T0226861

Common Pediatric Issues in Primary Care

Editors

LUZ M. FERNANDEZ
JONATHAN A. BECKER

PRIMARY CARE:
CLINICS IN OFFICE PRACTICE

www.primarycare.theclinics.com

Consulting Editor
JOEL J. HEIDELBAUGH

September 2021 • Volume 48 • Number 3

ELSEVIER

1600 John F. Kennedy Boulevard • Suite 1800 • Philadelphia, Pennsylvania, 19103-2899

http://www.theclinics.com

PRIMARY CARE: CLINICS IN OFFICE PRACTICE Volume 48, Number 3
September 2021 ISSN 0095-4543, ISBN-13: 978-0-323-79327-8

Editor: Katerina Heidhausen
Developmental Editor: Jessica Cañaberal

© 2021 Elsevier Inc. All rights reserved.

This periodical and the individual contributions contained in it are protected under copyright by Elsevier, and the following terms and conditions apply to their use:

Photocopying
Single photocopies of single articles may be made for personal use as allowed by national copyright laws. Permission of the Publisher and payment of a fee is required for all other photocopying, including multiple or systematic copying, copying for advertising or promotional purposes, resale, and all forms of document delivery. Special rates are available for educational institutions that wish to make photocopies for non-profit educational classroom use. For information on how to seek permission visit www.elsevier.com/permissions or call: (+44) 1865 843830 (UK)/(+1) 215 239 3804 (USA).

Derivative Works
Subscribers may reproduce tables of contents or prepare lists of articles including abstracts for internal circulation within their institutions. Permission of the Publisher is required for resale or distribution outside the institution. Permission of the Publisher is required for all other derivative works, including compilations and translations (please consult www.elsevier.com/permissions).

Electronic Storage or Usage
Permission of the Publisher is required to store or use electronically any material contained in this periodical, including any article or part of an article (please consult www.elsevier.com/permissions). Except as outlined above, no part of this publication may be reproduced, stored in a retrieval system or transmitted in any form or by any means, electronic, mechanical, photocopying, recording or otherwise, without prior written permission of the Publisher.

Notice
No responsibility is assumed by the Publisher for any injury and/or damage to persons or property as a matter of products liability, negligence or otherwise, or from any use or operation of any methods, products, instructions or ideas contained in the material herein. Because of rapid advances in the medical sciences, in particular, independent verification of diagnoses and drug dosages should be made.

Although all advertising material is expected to conform to ethical (medical) standards, inclusion in this publication does not constitute a guarantee or endorsement of the quality or value of such product or of the claims made of it by its manufacturer.

Primary Care: Clinics in Office Practice (ISSN: 0095-4543) is published quarterly by Elsevier Inc., 360 Park Avenue South, New York, NY 10010-1710. Months of issue are March, June, September, and December. Periodicals postage paid at New York, NY and additional mailing offices. Subscription prices are $261.00 per year (US individuals), $649.00 (US institutions), $100.00 (US students), $303.00 (Canadian individuals), $688.00 (Canadian institutions), $100.00 (Canadian students), $357.00 (international individuals), $688.00 (international institutions), and $175.00 (international students). Foreign air speed delivery is included in all *Clinics* subscription prices. All prices are subject to change without notice. POSTMASTER: Send address changes to *Primary Care: Clinics in Office Practice*, Elsevier Periodicals Customer Service, 11830 Westline Industrial Drive, St. Louis, MO 63146. Customer Service Health Sciences Division, Subscription Customer Service, 3251 Riverport Lane, Maryland Heights, MO 63043. **Customer Service: 1-800-654-2452 (U.S. and Canada); 314-447-8871 (outside U.S. and Canada). Fax: 314-447-8029. E-mail: journalscustomerservice-usa@elsevier.com (for print support); journalsonlinesupport-usa@elsevier.com (for online support).**

Reprints. For copies of 100 or more, of articles in this publication, please contact the Commercial Reprints Department, Elsevier Inc., 360 Park Avenue South, New York, NY 10010-1710. Tel. 212-633-3874; Fax: 212-633-3820; E-mail: reprints@elsevier.com.

Primary Care: Clinics in Office Practice is covered in *MEDLINE/PubMed (Index Medicus)* and *EMBASE/ Excerpta Medica, Current Contents/Clinical Medicine,* and *ISI/BIOMED.*

Contributors

CONSULTING EDITOR

JOEL J. HEIDELBAUGH, MD, FAAFP, FACG

Clinical Professor, Departments of Family Medicine and Urology, Director of Medical Student Education and Clerkship Director, Department of Family Medicine, University of Michigan Medical School, Ann Arbor, Michigan; Ypsilanti Health Center, Ypsilanti, Michigan

EDITORS

JONATHAN A. BECKER, MD

Chair, Department of Family and Geriatric Medicine, Professor, University of Louisville School of Medicine, Louisville, Kentucky

LUZ M. FERNANDEZ, MD

Program Director, Family Medicine Residency, Associate Professor, University of Louisville School of Medicine, Louisville, Kentucky

AUTHORS

NICOLE BICHIR, MD

Assistant Professor of Pediatrics, University of Louisville, Louisville, Kentucky

TINA FAWNS, MD

Assistant Professor, Department of Family and Community Medicine at the University of Kentucky, UK HealthCare: Turfland Medical Center, Lexington, Kentucky

CHRISTOPHER FOX, MD, CAQ-SM

Assistant Professor, University of Missouri-Kansas City, School of Medicine, Physician, Department of Community and Family Medicine, Truman Medical Centers, Kansas City, Missouri

MARGARET E. GIBSON, MD

Associate Professor, University of Missouri Kansas City, Department of Community and Family Medicine, Truman Medical Center Lakewood, Department of Orthopaedics and Musculoskeletal Medicine, Childrens Mercy Hospital, Kansas City, Missouri

KEVIN W. GRAY, MD, CAQ-SM, FAAFP

Assistant Professor, Department of Community and Family Medicine, Truman Medical Center Lakewood, Kansas City, Missouri

JORDAN HILGEFORT, MD, CAQSM

Assistant Professor, Department of Family and Geriatric Medicine, University of Louisville, Centers for Primary Care, Louisville, Kentucky

CAROL HUSTEDDE, PhD
Associate Professor, Department of Family and Community Medicine, University of Kentucky College of Medicine, Lexington, Kentucky

ASHLEY ILES, MD
Assistant Professor, Department of Family and Geriatric Medicine, University of Louisville, Louisville, Kentucky

SHERIDAN LANGFORD, MD
Assistant Professor of Pediatrics, University of Louisville, Louisville, Kentucky

MEGHANE E. MASQUELIN, DO
Resident, Family Medicine Residency Program, University of Louisville, Louisville, Kentucky

JEFFREY M. MEYER, MD
Assistant Professor of Pediatrics, University of Louisville, Louisville, Kentucky

ASHLEY E. NEAL, MD
Associate Professor, Department of Pediatrics, University of Louisville School of Medicine and Norton Children's, Louisville, Kentucky

JONATHAN NEWSOM, MD, CAQSM
Assistant Professor, Department of Family and Geriatric Medicine, University of Louisville, Centers for Primary Care, Louisville, Kentucky

KATHERINE M. POHLGEERS, MD
Assistant Professor, Department of Family Medicine and Geriatrics, University of Louisville, Louisville, Kentucky

AREZOO RAJAEE, MD
Resident, Department of Family Medicine and Geriatrics, University of Louisville, Louisville, Kentucky

BRITTNEY M. RICHARDSON, MD, CAQSM
Assistant Professor, Department of Family and Geriatric Medicine, University of Louisville, Louisville, Kentucky

MICHAEL SCOTT, DO
Pediatric Resident, Department of Pediatrics, University of Louisville, Office of Medical Education, School of Medicine, Louisville, Kentucky

NATALIE STORK, MD
Department of Orthopaedics and Musculoskeletal Medicine, Childrens Mercy Hospital, Assistant Professor, Orthopaedic Surgery, University of Missouri-Kansas City School of Medicine, Kansas City, Missouri

NEENA THOMAS-EAPEN, MD, FAAFP
Associate Professor, Clinical Track, College of Medicine, University of Kentucky, Lexington, Kentucky

Contents

> Most children with congenital heart disease (CHD) survive to adulthood, owing largely to significant advances in the diagnosis and management of CHD over the past few decades. Primary care providers are essential partners in the recognition and management of these patients in our current medical environment. This article reviews the role of the primary care physician in detecting fetuses, infants, and children with possible CHD. Furthermore, this article discusses common primary care issues arising for patients with CHD, including growth and development, mental illness, dental care, and the transition to adult primary care.

> Pediatric hypertension is becoming of increasing concern as the incidence rate increases alongside pediatric obesity. Practitioners need to be aware of the screening recommendations for early recognition and management of this disorder. Lifestyle modifications should be addressed early and specialty referral considered if the child is not improving. Further work-up to rule out secondary causes of pediatric hypertension should also be considered in any child with stage 2 hypertension and in those with persistently elevated blood pressures. Early recognition and management are key to not only preventing present complications but also future cardiovascular disease in adulthood.

> In the pediatric population, asthma is the most common chronic disease. Asthma is a chronic inflammatory disease consisting of variable respiratory symptoms and airflow limitation. Proper and timely diagnosis remains of utmost importance. Early diagnosis allows for earlier treatment and subsequent reduction of morbidity and mortality. Newer research and medications have changed the treatment paradigm, including the addition of biologic agents for more severe cases and use of inhaled corticosteroid–formoterol inhaler as a rescue treatment.

Video content accompanies this article at http://www.primarycare. theclinics.com.

As a child matures so does the child's gait pattern. Gait changes in pediatric patients will be expected and sequential as developmental milestones. Gait changes may also represent normal variations along an appropriate spectrum. There are times when changes in gait are due to urgent orthopedic or medical conditions, and those should not be overlooked. A good understanding of pediatric gait development and a basic understanding of gait assessment are critical for the primary care physician who cares for children.

This article reviews injuries encountered in active pediatric patients and discusses common presentations, diagnostic criteria, treatment modalities, and prevention. An emphasis is placed on overuse injuries, including a review of physeal and apophyseal injuries encountered in skeletally immature, active patients as well as back disorders often encountered in adolescents. This article is not meant to be comprehensive, but it offers directions for management of these patients in the outpatient primary care setting.

This article reviews common issues in pediatric dental health, including normal development, developmental issues, infections, trauma, and preventative care.

There is arguably no group of conditions more common and expansive in children than gastrointestinal disorders. Moreover, successful recognition, diagnosis, and management of these ailments is particularly challenging provided the breadth of potential dysfunction, as well as a general paucity of specific physical examination findings to pinpoint diagnoses. Elucidation of these conditions is made further challenging by frequent difficulty of pediatric patients to provide a detailed articulation of their symptoms. Nonetheless, a thorough history can aid in distinguishing these various diagnoses, which can be further classified into 3 categories: infectious, inflammatory, and immunologic pathology; motility disorders; and functional gastrointestinal disorders

This article describes the current understanding of the identification, classification, and diagnosis of autism spectrum disorder (ASD) as it relates to the practice of primary care providers. In addition, the most updated information regarding risk factors, as well as effective treatment strategies are provided. Although primary care providers are not typically the experts in ASD treatment, they constitute a critical component of the care team responsible for early identification and intervention initiation for patients with ASD.

The treatment of attention-deficit/hyperactivity disorder can be a very rewarding and challenging task. The management of this condition has impact on a child's performance in school in both academics and extracurriculars, and therefore, can be a determinant of what they are able to achieve and become. Treatment can also impact the child's self-image and ability to successfully interact with their peers. Adequate control of the disorder can break down barriers to successful development of a child's potential and ability to play a role in the work force someday.

Adverse childhood experiences are found in adults regardless of race, socioeconomic level, or education. They can be identified in a clinical environment by answering a retrospective questionnaire . Adverse childhood experiences are clearly linked to high-risk health behaviors and multiple chronic diseases. Extensive knowledge exists about the severe impact of adverse childhood experiences in adults. Identification efforts have begun for children showing the prevalence and categories of abuse. National surveillance surveys capture prevalence data for children at the state level. The for Disease Control and Prevention has distributed prevention strategies to decrease the likelihood of adverse childhood experiences in children.

Childhood obesity is a pathologic process with multifactorial causes. The reasons range widely. Obesity leads to chronic health conditions, increasing morbidity. The management of obesity must include the patient, family, school, community, and even government for policy changes. Lifestyle changes are the mainstay of treatment, including a healthy diet and increased physical activity. Medications and bariatric surgery may have a role in certain severe cases. Community and policy changes concerning food and physical activities may facilitate practical strategies against the increasing obesity epidemic. It will help families and health care systems tackle childhood obesity effectively.

Allergy is a broad topic encompassing common clinical allergic diseases, asthma, and complex immunodeficiencies. In this article, the authors discuss the most common allergic diseases and anaphylaxis and briefly review the current knowledge and management of food allergies, allergic rhinitis, otitis media, sinusitis, chronic cough, atopic dermatitis, urticarial and angioedema, contact dermatitis, allergic ophthalmopathy, drug allergy, latex allergy, and insect sting. Because the prevalence of allergic disorders continues to increase, it is increasingly important for physicians to stay up to date on most recent evidence-based diagnosis and management of allergic disorders.

PRIMARY CARE:
CLINICS IN OFFICE PRACTICE

SERIES OF RELATED INTEREST

Medical Clinics (http://www.medical.theclinics.com)
Physician Assistant Clinics (https://www.physicianassistant.theclinics.com)

THE CLINICS ARE AVAILABLE ONLINE!
Access your subscription at:
www.theclinics.com

Foreword
Meeting Children's Greatest Needs

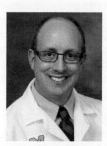

Joel J. Heidelbaugh, MD, FAAFP, FACG
Consulting Editor

The COVID-19 pandemic has brought many challenges to all of us, especially to our pediatric patients and our own children. This last academic year was either mostly or entirely virtual, certainly not optimal, and the forward academic progression for many children was hampered. Social isolation prevented gatherings, school activities, and even playing outside in the neighborhood. We will likely not fully understand the ramifications and impact of the pandemic on our children for years to come. Moreover, it has been a challenge for many of our pediatric patients to get the health care they deserve and need. Access to care has suffered; children have fallen behind in immunizations and routine well child care, while the need for attention to address and treat mental health and disorders and developmental delay has never been greater. Such is the case with most things in life; the opportunities are unfortunately not equal for everyone.

So how do we eliminate racial, ethnic, and socioeconomic disparities in the health care of our children, especially during a pandemic with no short term end in sight? How do we identify and meet the greatest needs of our pediatric patients at a time when access to health care is limited and resources are strained? A brilliant and provocative article in *The Lancet* posits[1] that we need to ask tougher questions, and that research must encompass all racial groups and multiracial children while ending a classification of "*racial and ethnic disparities as mere social determinants issues given evidence to the contrary.*" The article highlights that "*much more emphasis should be placed on evaluating and disseminating evidence-based interventions that actually eliminate disparities,*" including parent mentors who have children with a certain health condition and are trained to help other parents and children with the same condition. This intervention has been shown to decrease health care costs through fewer emergency department visits and hospitalizations, to improve overall access to health care, to provide more children with sustainable medical insurance, and to achieve greater

Prim Care Clin Office Pract 48 (2021) xi–xii
https://doi.org/10.1016/j.pop.2021.05.001
0095-4543/21/© 2021 Published by Elsevier Inc.

child and parent satisfaction and quality of care while reducing and eliminating disparities.

I would like to acknowledge and thank our guest editors for this issue of *Primary Care: Clinics in Office Practice*, Dr Luz Fernandez and Dr Jonathan Becker, for their diligent efforts in creating the vision for this important collection of articles on relevant pediatric topics in primary care. This formidable effort was conceived and completed during a year when health care providers have been overworked, overstressed, and yet they still give often more than they have. The issue highlights pediatric cardiac, pulmonary, neurologic, orthopedic, and gastrointestinal conditions, allergies and anaphylaxis, autism and attention deficit disorders, obesity management, adverse childhood experiences, and dental care. This was truly an outstanding effort by all our author experts, as they highlighted key evidence-based provisions of care and addressed key social determinants and barriers to effective health care in our children. I hope that our readers find this issue to be as informative and educational as I have.

Joel J. Heidelbaugh, MD, FAAFP, FACG
Departments of Family Medicine and Urology
University of Michigan Medical School
Ann Arbor, MI, USA

Ypsilanti Health Center
200 Arnet Suite 200
Ypsilanti, MI 48198, USA

E-mail address:
jheidel@umich.edu

REFERENCE

1. Flores G, Hollenbach JP, Hogan AH. To eliminate racial and ethnic disparities in child health care, more needs to be addressed than just social determinants. Lancet 2019;7(10):842–3.

Preface

Common Pediatric Issues in Primary Care: An Introduction

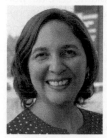 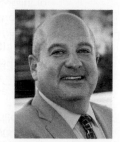

Luz M. Fernandez, MD   Jonathan A. Becker, MD
Editors

The goal of this issue has been to create an easy reference for some of the most common pediatric issues that are encountered in the primary care setting. It is our hope that the reader can utilize the knowledge gained here to better manage these pediatric-specific problems with current and evidence-based recommendations, whether it be through therapeutics, testing, or referrals. We have concentrated on areas the clinician will encounter frequently in a typical practice. These encompass cardiac, pulmonary, musculoskeletal, dental, and gastrointestinal systems. Further articles are then dedicated to some of the psychiatric issues that have become increasingly recognized in this population, such as autism spectrum disorders, attention deficit issues, and the impact of adverse childhood events. Articles are also dedicated to pediatric obesity, which is present in epidemic proportions, as well as allergy and anaphylaxis.

We can't thank the authors and editors enough for their hard work in putting these articles together. The vast majority of the work was done amidst the COVID-19 pandemic that placed a multitude of stressors on the contributors to this work. Our appreciation to the collaborators from a number of departments at the University of Louisville, the Department of Family and Community Medicine at the University of

Prim Care Clin Office Pract 48 (2021) xiii–xiv
https://doi.org/10.1016/j.pop.2021.05.002
0095-4543/21/© 2021 Published by Elsevier Inc.   **primarycare.theclinics.com**

Kentucky, and the Department of Community and Family Medicine at the University of Missouri–Kansas City.

Luz M. Fernandez, MD
Department of Family and Geriatric Medicine
University of Louisville
501 East Broadway, Suite 270
Louisville, KY 40202, USA

Jonathan A. Becker, MD
Department of Family and Geriatric Medicine
University of Louisville
501 East Broadway, Suite 270
Louisville, KY 40202, USA

E-mail addresses:
luz.fernandez@louisville.edu (L.M. Fernandez)
jon.becker@louisville.edu (J.A. Becker)

Congenital Heart Disease

Michael Scott, DO[a], Ashley E. Neal, MD[b],*

KEYWORDS

- Congenital heart disease • Pediatric cardiology • CHD • Screening
- Patent ductus arteriosus

KEY POINTS

- Most children with congenital heart disease (CHD) survive to adulthood.
- The genetic cause of CHD continues to be elucidated; thus, consultation with a pediatric geneticist or pediatric cardiologist may be useful in children with genetic syndromes when the cardiac implications are unclear.
- Because the availability and accuracy of prenatal screening for certain cardiac lesions varies, pediatricians must remain vigilant for neonates presenting with symptoms that suggest CHD.
- Children with CHD need comprehensive pediatric care that considers the increased risk of growth issues, developmental delay, and mental health disorders in this population.

INTRODUCTION

Congenital heart disease (CHD) is the most common birth defect, affecting 8 to 10 per 1000 newborns in the United States and 17.9 per 1000 newborns worldwide. Fortunately, the mortality rate for CHD has decreased by 34.5% globally between 1990 and 2017, due largely to rapid advances in diagnostic imaging, medications, catheter techniques, and surgical interventions.[1] Recent estimates suggest about 2.4 million adults in the United States and 12 million adults globally are survivors of CHD.[1,2] For children with CHD, the pediatric primary care provider and pediatric cardiologist collaborate to identify CHD, monitor for symptoms, counsel about necessary interventions, and ultimately provide optimal transitions to adult providers. These children, who often have multiple comorbidities, receive the best care through a team-based approach coordinated by the primary care physician, establishing a medical home.[3]

[a] Department of Pediatrics, University of Louisville, Office of Medical Education, School of Medicine, 571 South Floyd, Suite 412, Louisville, KY 40202, USA; [b] Department of Pediatrics, University of Louisville School of Medicine and Norton Children's, 571 South Floyd Street, Suite 113, Louisville, KY 40202, USA
* Corresponding author.
E-mail address: ashley.neal.1@louisville.edu

Prim Care Clin Office Pract 48 (2021) 351–366
https://doi.org/10.1016/j.pop.2021.04.005
0095-4543/21/© 2021 Elsevier Inc. All rights reserved.

primarycare.theclinics.com

CAUSE OF CONGENITAL HEART DISEASE

The cause of CHD is multifactorial with both environmental and genetic influences. Thus, it is useful for primary care providers, geneticists, obstetricians, and pediatric cardiologists to have a basic understanding of these risk factors. Although the association between genetic factors and CHD was first recognized in the late 1940s, the precise relationship between specific genetic mutations and CHD remains quite complex.[4] Rarely, a single gene has been linked to a specific lesion. More frequently, genetic syndromes are associated with a diverse array of cardiac lesions as shown in **Table 1**.[4] New genes correlated with CHD or cardiomyopathy continue to be identified on a regular basis, making the rote memorization of all genes potentially associated with cardiac pathology an impossible undertaking. It would be practical to reference Online Mendelian Inheritance in Man (OMIM)[5] or consult a pediatric geneticist or pediatric cardiologist when a genetic abnormality or syndrome is suspected and the cardiac implications are unclear. Many congenital heart defects are identified prenatally, with one indication for a fetal echocardiogram being suspicion of a genetic condition by cell-free fetal DNA testing.[6] Environmental risk factors also contribute to the development of CHD. Reported prenatal risk factors include maternal ingestion of ethanol or prescription medications such as sodium valproate, retinoic acid, lithium, nonsteroidal antiinflammatory drugs, angiotensin-converting enzyme inhibitors, and paroxetine. During pregnancy, maternal infections such as rubella and cytomegalovirus and poorly controlled maternal diabetes are also well-described environmental risk factors associated with subsequent development of CHD.[6,7] Environmental risk factors may also prompt referral for fetal echocardiogram and subsequent prenatal detection of CHD (**Table 2**).

PRENATAL DIAGNOSIS OF CONGENITAL HEART DISEASE

The care of many children with CHD begins prenatally with maternal referral for a fetal echocardiogram. Referral may be based on findings from the obstetric evaluation or other predisposing conditions as noted in **Table 2**. This testing is considered cost-effective when risk of CHD exceeds 3%.[6] Comprehensive fetal echocardiograms, which often include additional views of cardiac structures and color Doppler imaging, can increase detection rates of CHD from less than 50% to nearly 90% of serious CHD when compared with routine obstetric ultrasounds.[6,8–10] When CHD is identified prenatally, families can receive appropriate counseling and delivery plans can be adjusted accordingly, reducing preoperative mortality.[11] Unfortunately, even within the United States, large disparities exist in prenatal detection of CHD, with diagnosis rates among states ranging from 11.8% to 53.4%.[12] Remote interpretation of fetal echocardiograms coupled with sonographer training can improve prenatal CHD detection rates. However, this strategy has only been implemented in limited regions of the country.[13] Therefore, normal prenatal assessments do not exclude structural heart disease. Even when a comprehensive fetal echocardiogram has been performed, some aspects of the fetal circulation differ from the postnatal circulation, limiting the diagnostic accuracy of fetal examinations for certain lesions. For example, a patent ductus arteriosus (PDA) would be a normal finding during fetal life. Therefore, predicting whether or not a child will develop heart failure from a PDA postnatally is nearly impossible based on prenatal imaging.

NORMAL FETAL AND TRANSITIONAL CIRCULATION

During fetal life, most of the gas exchange occurs at the placenta, with only 10% to 25% of the blood ejected by the right ventricle making it to the fetal lungs.[14] The

Table 1
Examples of genetic syndromes commonly associated with cardiac disease

Genetic Syndrome [associated gene(s)]	Extracardiac Features	Associated Cardiac Disease
Trisomy 21	Brachycephaly, small ears, upslanting palpebral fissures, epicanthal folds, duodenal atresia, imperforate anus, Hirschsprung disease, leukemia	AVSD, VSD, ASD, PDA, TOF, pulmonary hypertension
Trisomy 18	Micrognathia, short sternum, rocker-bottom feet, omphalocele, renal anomalies, severe intellectual disability	ASD, VSD, PDA, TOF, DORV, TGA, valve abnormalities
Trisomy 13	Cleft lip and palate, hypotelorism, coloboma, holoprosencephaly, deafness, severe intellectual disability, polydactyly, omphalocele, cryptorchidism	ASD, VSD, PDA, valve abnormalities
Turner syndrome	Short stature, early loss of ovarian function, lymphedema, webbed neck, renal anomalies	Coarctation of the aorta, aortic stenosis, BAV
CHARGE syndrome (CHD7, SEMA3E)	Coloboma, choanal atresia, genital hypoplasia, ear abnormalities, hearing loss, developmental delay, growth retardation, intellectual disability	ASD, VSD, TOF
DiGeorge syndrome, velocardiofacial syndrome (TBX1)	Myopathic facies, tubular nose with bulbous nasal tip, immunodeficiency, hypocalcemia, intellectual disability	TOF, IAA, TA, VSD
Holt-Oram syndrome (TBX5)	Absent thumb, radius hypoplasia/limb defects, triphalangeal thumb	ASD, VSD, PDA, AVSD, conduction defects
Alagille syndrome (JAGGED1, NOTCH2)	Prominent forehead, hypertelorism, intellectual disability, liver failure, ophthalmologic problems, butterfly vertebrae, renal defects	Peripheral pulmonary stenosis, PS, TOF
Noonan syndrome (PTPN11, KRAS, SOS1, SOS2, RAF1, BRAF, MEK1, HRAS, NRAS, SHOC2, CBL, NF1)	Short stature, hypertelorism, ptosis, pectus deformity, bleeding disorder, chylothorax, cryptorchidism, lymphatic abnormalities	PS, ASD, TOF, VSD, PDA, hypertrophic cardiomyopathy

(continued on next page)

Table 1
(continued)

Genetic Syndrome [associated gene(s)]	Extracardiac Features	Associated Cardiac Disease
Williams syndrome (ELN)	Short stature, flat midface, epicanthal folds, long philtrum, sensorineural hearing loss, thick lips, intellectual disability, sociable, hypercalcemia	Supravalvular AS, peripheral PS, VSD, ASD
Marfan Syndrome (Fibrillin)	Arm span to height >1.05, disproportionate tall stature, long narrow face, ectopia lentis, pectus excavatum, pectus carinatum, high-arched palate	Aortic aneurysm, mitral valve prolapse, dilated pulmonary artery
Kabuki syndrome (KMT2D, KDM6A)	Growth deficiency, wide palpebral fissure, intellectual disability, fetal finger pads	ASD, VSD, TOF, coarctation of aorta, BAV, TGA, HLHS
Ellis-van Creveld (EVC, EVC2)	Short upper lip, natal teeth, enamel hypoplasia, polydactyly	ASD, common atrium

Abbreviations: AS, aortic stenosis; ASD, atrial septal defect; AVSD, atrioventricular septal defect; BAV, bicuspid aortic valve; DORV, double outlet right ventricle; HLHS, hypoplastic left heart syndrome; IAA, interrupted aortic arch; PDA, patent ductus arteriosus; PS, pulmonary stenosis; TA, truncus arteriosus; TGA, transposition of the great arteries; TOF, tetralogy of Fallot; VSD, ventricular septal defect.
Data from Refs.[4,5,15]

Table 2
Indications for fetal echocardiogram

Screening Indicated	May be Considered	Not Indicated
Maternal Indications		
• Uncontrolled (Hgb A1C >6) pregestational diabetes mellitus (DM) • DM diagnosed in 1st trimester • Uncontrolled phenylketonuria • Anti-Ro (SSA)/anti-La (SSB)+ autoantibodies with a previously affected child • Retinoic acid use (third trimester) • Nonsteroidal antiinflammatory drug (NSAID) use (third trimester) • ubella (first trimester)	• Anti-Ro (SSA)/anti-La (SSB)+ autoantibodies without a previously affected child • Angiotensin-converting enzyme inhibitor use • Anticonvulsant use • Lithium use • Vitamin A use • Paroxetine use • NSAIDs (first/second trimester) • Pregnancy resulting from assisted reproduction technology	• Gestational DM with Hgb A1c <6% • Vitamin K agonist use • Selective serotonin reuptake inhibitor use (other than paroxetine) • Maternal infection other than rubella with seroconversion only
Fetal Indications		
• Suspected fetal cardiac abnormality by obstetric ultrasound • Extracardiac abnormality identified by obstetric ultrasound • Infection with suspicion of fetal myocarditis • Suspected or confirmed chromosome abnormality • Fetal tachycardia, bradycardia, or frequent or persistent irregular heart rhythm • Increased nuchal thickness >99% (≥3.5 mm) • Increased nuchal thickness >95% (≥3 mm) with abnormal ductus venosus flow • Monochorionic twinning • Fetal hydrops or effusions	• Increased nuchal thickness >95% (≥3 mm) • Abnormality of the umbilical cord • Abnormality of the placenta • Abnormality of intraabdominal venous anatomy	

(continued on next page)

Table 2
(continued)

Screening Indicated	May be Considered	Not Indicated
Family History		
• CHD in 1st degree relative of the fetus • Relative with disorder with mendelian inheritance that has a CHD association	CHD in a second degree relative of the fetus	Isolated CHD in a relative other than first or second degree

Data from Donofrio MT, Moon-Grady AJ, Hornberger LK et al. American Heart Association Adults With Congenital Heart Disease Joint Committee of the Council on Cardiovascular Disease in the Young and Council on Clinical Cardiology, Council on Cardiovascular Surgery and Anesthesia, and Council on Cardiovascular and Stroke Nursing. Diagnosis and treatment of fetal cardiac disease: a scientific statement from the American Heart Association. Circulation. 2014 May 27;129(21):2183-242.

PDA allows blood oxygenated in the placenta to travel from the pulmonary artery to the descending aorta, bypassing the fetal lungs.[14–16] During fetal life, pulmonary vascular resistance (PVR) is elevated, leading to right-to-left shunting at the PDA. Following delivery of the newborn, oxygen tension increases, and the newborn lungs expand, forcing amniotic fluid from the alveolar sacs. These changes dramatically decrease the PVR, which combined with a concomitant increase in the systemic vascular resistance, results in shunting across the PDA becoming left-to-right (from the aorta to the pulmonary artery). The PDA begins to functionally close at approximately 10 to 15 hours of life and is anatomically closed by around 2 to 3 weeks in most infants in response to persistently increased arterial oxygen tension and decreased prostaglandin (PGE) levels.[14] Over the first 6 to 8 weeks of life, the PVR continues to decrease to normal adult levels.[15] These physiologic changes are important to consider when evaluating a patient with confirmed or suspected CHD as will be discussed in subsequent sections.

PULSE OXIMETRY SCREENING

Acknowledging the limitations of prenatal testing and dynamic aspects of neonatal cardiovascular physiology, providers caring for newborns must remain vigilant for children who develop signs or symptoms that may suggest CHD. In conjunction with a comprehensive history and physical examination, predischarge pulse oximetry has an overall sensitivity of 76.3% and specificity of 99.9% in detecting critical CHD.[17–19] This screening should be performed no sooner than 24 hours of life and, ideally, as close to newborn nursery discharge as possible. For this assessment, oxygen saturation is measured in the right arm and a foot. When the oxygen saturation is greater than or equal to 95% in either the right arm or a foot with less than or equal to 3% difference between measured saturations, no additional screening is indicated. Otherwise, the infant requires repeat pulse oximetry measurement. With persistently abnormal findings, noncardiac causes of hypoxia ought to be excluded. In the absence of a noncardiac cause of hypoxia, the child should undergo a pediatric echocardiogram to evaluate for CHD.[18,20]

NEONATAL PRESENTATIONS OF CONGENITAL HEART DISEASE

The timing and symptomatology of neonatal presentations of CHD can best be understood in the context of the physiologic changes that occur with the transition from fetal to postnatal life (**Fig. 1**). Some of the more common forms of CHD, emphasizing key physical examination findings and lesions that may require intervention, are briefly discussed.

NEONATAL CONGENITAL HEART DISEASE REQUIRING EMERGENT INTERVENTION
Total Anomalous Pulmonary Venous Return

- Brief overview: the connection of all 4 pulmonary veins is abnormal and/or obstructed.
- Presentation: may develop cyanosis, respiratory distress, and symptoms of low cardiac output within the first few hours of life, as newborn lung perfusion increases significantly.
- Treatment: urgent surgical correction

This is one of the few surgical emergencies in pediatric cardiology. Importantly, it is also a lesion in which PGE may cause further deterioration by increasing pulmonary blood flow, worsening pulmonary edema. Children most at risk for decompensation

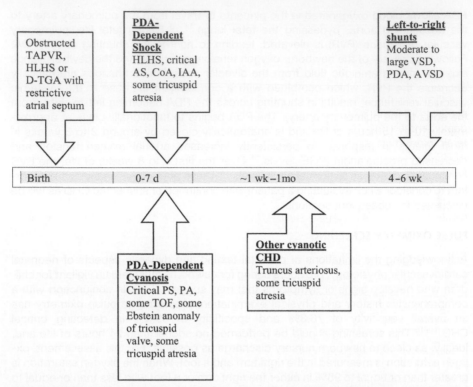

Fig. 1. Neonatal presentations of CHD. AS, aortic stenosis; ASD, atrial septal defect; AVSD, atrioventricular septal defect; CoA, coarctation; D-TGA, D-transposition of the great arteries; HLHS, hypoplastic left heart syndrome; IAA, interrupted aortic arch; PA, pulmonary atresia; PDA, patent ductus arteriosus; PS, pulmonary stenosis; TAPVR, Total anomalous pulmonary venous return; TOF, tetralogy of Fallot; VSD, ventricular septal defect.

with this lesion have infracardiac total anomalous pulmonary venous return (TAPVR), in which the pulmonary venous return travels through the liver. Of note, in the absence of pulmonary venous obstruction, infants with TAPVR may have minimal symptoms.[21,22]

D-Transposition of the Great Arteries

- Brief overview: systemic and pulmonary circulation occur in parallel with the aorta arising from the right ventricle and the pulmonary artery from the left ventricle.
- Presentation: may present either at birth or in the first few days of life with variable degree of cyanosis, may develop acidosis
- Treatment: PGE; may need urgent balloon atrial septostomy

In D-transposition of the great arteries (D-TGA), although the PDA may permit some oxygenated blood to reach the body, a minimally restrictive atrial level shunt is required to adequately support the systemic circulation. Children with D-TGA and restrictive atrial septal defects (ASDs) may present either at birth or in the first few days of life with profound cyanosis and acidosis, requiring an emergent interventional cardiology procedure called a balloon atrial septostomy to enlarge the ASD. Children with adequate atrial mixing may have mild-to-moderate cyanosis at birth and typically require PGE until definitive surgical repair is performed in the first week of life.[22,23]

Hypoplastic Left Heart Syndrome

- Brief overview: mitral valve, left ventricle, and aorta do not develop appropriately
- Presentation: may develop signs of respiratory distress and low cardiac output, may have cyanosis
- Treatment: PGE; may need urgent balloon atrial septostomy

Although not technically a form of cyanotic CHD, infants with hypoplastic left heart syndrome (HLHS) often exhibit cyanosis due to requisite mixing of oxygenated and deoxygenated blood. In this lesion, mixing at the ASD is necessary to support the systemic blood flow due to the severe hypoplasia of left-sided heart structures. Thus, HLHS is another lesion in which a balloon atrial septostomy may be needed in the first few hours to days of life if a restrictive ASD is present. Infants with HLHS can develop signs of respiratory distress and low cardiac output from either ductal constriction or restrictive ASDs. Therefore, these infants also require PGE until the first stage of surgical palliation called the Norwood procedure is performed.[24–26]

DUCTAL-DEPENDENT LESIONS NOT REQUIRING EMERGENT INTERVENTION

Several lesions in the newborn period require the PDA to support either the systemic or pulmonary blood flow but do not typically need emergent intervention (**Table 3**). Many children with ductal-dependent pulmonary blood flow will have cyanosis evident

Table 3
Ductal-dependent lesions not requiring emergent intervention

	[a]Ductal-Dependent Pulmonary Blood Flow	[a]Ductal-Dependent Systemic Blood Flow
Lesion and Key Points	**Critical pulmonary stenosis (PS)** • Loud murmur • +PGE	**Hypoplastic left heart syndrome (HLHS)** • May require emergent intervention • Requires unrestrictive ASD and PDA • +PGE
	Pulmonary atresia • +PGE	**Critical aortic stenosis** • Loud murmur • +PGE
	Tetralogy of Fallot (TOF), some forms • Loud murmur • Cyanosis may be progressive/risk for "Tet" spells • +/−PGE • Consider 22q11 testing	**Critical coarctation of the aorta (CoA)** • More likely to be missed with pulse oximetry screen • May present with shock first week of life • +PGE
	Ebstein anomaly of tricuspid valve (severe forms) • Loud murmur • Marked cardiomegaly on chest radiograph • +/−PGE	**Interrupted aortic arch** • More likely to be missed with pulse oximetry screen • May present with shock first week of life • +PGE • Consider 22q11 testing
	Tricuspid atresia (some forms) • +/−PGE	**Tricuspid atresia (some forms)** • May present with shock first week of life if VSD restrictive • +/−PGE

Abbreviations: ASD, atrial septal defect; PDA, patent ductus arteriosus; PGE, prostaglandin; VSD, ventricular septal defect.
[a] See notes in text regarding decision-making related to initiation of PGE in these lesions.

clinically or by pulse oximetry in the first hours to days of life. Although some lesions in this category will require PGE until an intervention is performed, close monitoring for development of marked cyanosis with PDA closure may be needed to determine whether other lesions are truly ductal dependent. It is worth noting that infants with tetralogy of Fallot (TOF) are at risk for the development of progressive subpulmonary stenosis. This subpulmonary stenosis usually worsens at a few months of age, creating a substrate for hypercyanotic episodes or "tetralogy spells." In these episodes, the infant's murmur may become inaudible due to a significant decrement in pulmonary blood flow as deoxygenated blood flows right to left across the ventricular septal defect and out the aorta. To abort episodes, the infant should be soothed, given oxygen, and the knees pushed toward the chest among other maneuvers to favor pulmonary over systemic blood flow. Once hypercyanotic episodes have been observed, an infant with TOF warrants urgent surgical intervention.[27,28]

Lesions that require the PDA to support systemic blood flow (see **Table 3**) may not be adequately identified by prenatal ultrasound or newborn pulse oximetry and may present in shock with ductal closure in the first week of life.[29] Thus, one should have a high index of suspicion for possible ductal-dependent CHD in the neonate presenting with shock in the first few weeks of life and a low threshold for initiation of PGE. Although tricuspid atresia is considered a form of cyanotic CHD, it is a complex lesion that presents with a variable degree of cyanosis and can present with shock if systemic blood flow becomes compromised due to a restrictive ventricular septal defect.[27,30]

OTHER NEONATAL CONGENITAL HEART DISEASE PRESENTATIONS
"Cyanotic" Congenital Heart Disease: Tricuspid Atresia and Truncus Arteriosus

Tricuspid atresia is a highly variable and complex, cyanotic single ventricle CHD lesion. Some infants with this lesion require PGE to maintain pulmonary or systemic blood flow depending on the relative position of the great vessels (eg, D-transposition). Other infants with tricuspid atresia, normal position of the great arteries, and a large ventricular septal defect will develop pulmonary edema over the first few weeks of life and may require a surgical procedure called a pulmonary artery band to restrict pulmonary blood flow if they develop tachypnea, tiring with feeds, sweating with feeds, and poor growth that suggest heart failure.[27,30] Truncus arteriosus is another CHD lesion typically included with cyanotic CHD lesions due to obligate mixing of oxygenated and deoxygenated blood at an unrestrictive ventricular septal defect and a single outflow supplying the body and lungs. However, many infants with truncus arteriosus will have nearly normal oxygen saturations. Clinically, children with this lesion usually develop pulmonary edema, tachypnea, and signs of heart failure within the first few weeks of life.[27]

Left-To-Right Shunts

As the PVR normalizes over the first 6 to 8 weeks of life, infants with moderate-to-large left-to-right shunts develop symptoms of pulmonary overcirculation. This category includes infants with a ventricular septal defect, atrioventricular canal defect, patent ductus arteriosus, or ASD. However, ASDs rarely cause symptoms in infancy. Infants with significant left-to-right shunts may initially be asymptomatic, have soft murmurs with large ventricular septal defects, or have more obvious murmurs with some large PDAs. However, in the first 1 to 2 months of life, these infants may demonstrate a gradual decline in growth percentiles or develop progressive tachypnea, worsening reflux, sweating with feeds, and/or tiring with feeds. These symptoms of heart failure may respond to increased caloric intake and initiation of diuretics, but consultation with a pediatric cardiologist is recommended. In contrast, many types of asymptomatic CHD are also identified in the neonatal period. For example, infants with small, isolated ventricular septal defects may have readily apparent murmurs prompting evaluation, but these defects would not be expected to cause symptoms and may spontaneously resolve in the first few years of life. In addition, mild valve abnormalities or dysfunction (ie, bicuspid aortic valve) may also be identified during the newborn period.[31]

Childhood Presentations of Congenital Heart Disease

Many types of CHD requiring intervention are recognized in newborns. During childhood and adolescence, pediatric cardiologists often see children for acquired forms of heart disease such as Kawasaki disease and cardiomyopathy or nonstructural concerns such as arrhythmia. Two relatively common CHD lesions presenting in childhood or adolescence are ASD and noncritical CoA. Although ASDs are generally asymptomatic, many are diagnosed incidentally as part of a murmur evaluation. Careful auscultation in children with these lesions may demonstrate a fixed, split S2 or pulmonary flow murmur. An electrocardiogram may demonstrate right axis deviation or right ventricular hypertrophy. A high index of suspicion is needed for detection of this lesion because symptoms and physical examination findings may be subtle.[32] One should consider expert consultation for additional diagnostic testing if an abnormality is suspected by physical examination or electrocardiogram. Noncritical CoA, in which patency of the ductus arteriosus is not required to maintain cardiac output, becomes evident in childhood or adolescence. Children with noncritical CoA may have upper-extremity hypertension, femoral pulses occurring after radial pulses (radial-femoral delay), intermittent claudication, or a systolic murmur at the left lower sternal border radiating to the back.[25,26] Thus, in children with hypertension, blood pressure in all 4 extremities and femoral pulses should be assessed.

LONGITUDINAL FOLLOW-UP ISSUES IN THE CHILD WITH CONGENITAL HEART DISEASE
Growth and Development

The child with CHD may have associated anomalies or comorbidities related to chronic illness, prior interventions, and prolonged hospitalizations. Approximately, 25% of infants with CHD have a noncardiac anomaly and about 15% have multiple congenital anomalies.[7] Those caring for children with CHD should have a low threshold to obtain genetic testing or consultation as well as diagnostic tests to evaluate for extracardiac comorbidities. Understanding whether or not a genetic abnormality is present may help determine the likelihood and expected magnitude of developmental delay (DD), which might be seen for the child.

Factors in children with CHD that increase risk of DD are as follows[33,34]:

- History of heart surgery in infancy
- Cyanotic lesions not requiring open heart surgery
- Premature birth
- Known genetic anomaly associated with DD
- History of mechanical support (ie, extracorporeal membrane oxygenation or ventricular assist device)
- History of heart transplantation
- History of cardiopulmonary resuscitation
- History of prolonged hospitalization (>2 weeks)

- Perioperative seizures
- Significant abnormalities on brain imaging

Any child or adolescent with CHD and developmental concern should be referred for formal developmental evaluation to optimize neurodevelopmental outcomes and quality of life.[33,34] In addition to developmental concerns, growth issues in infants and children with CHD are prevalent. In early childhood, even children with nonsurgical and repaired CHD may demonstrate poor relative growth.[35] However, in later childhood, rates of combined obesity and overweight in children with CHD mirror the general population at about 29%.[36] Some parents may restrict physical activity inappropriately in a child with repaired CHD or continue to provide excess calories when supplementation is not needed.[36] Thus, children with CHD may need specific counseling about physical activity and nutrition throughout childhood and adolescence. Overweight and obese children with CHD, as all children, require screening for development of associated comorbidities such as hypertension, diabetes, obstructive sleep apnea, and nonalcoholic fatty liver disease.[35]

Mental Illness

As noted earlier, children with CHD are at increased risk for developmental delay, specifically issues with executive function and attention, which may predispose them to subsequent development of mental illness in adolescence and adulthood.[37] In a recent Colorado statewide survey, 20% of adolescents with CHD had mental illness including anxiety disorders, attention disorders, conduct disorders, and impulse control disorders. Not surprisingly, those with a genetic diagnosis and a higher number of recent cardiac procedures had an increased risk of mental illness.[38] When evaluating adolescent CHD patients with single ventricle lesions, the lifetime risk of psychiatric diagnosis was ~65%, with anxiety disorders and attention disorders seen most frequently.[39] Thus, screening and addressing any psychiatric comorbidity in this population is crucial to improving overall quality of life and general well-being.

Dental Care

Another important aspect of primary care for children with CHD, as other pediatric patients, is encouraging routine dental visits. Although CHD is a known risk factor for developing infective endocarditis, recent guidelines suggest only a limited number of high-risk lesions require antibiotic prophylaxis before invasive dental procedures.[40] Children who need prophylaxis include those with

- Prosthetic cardiac valve or valve material,
- Previous endocarditis,
- Unrepaired or palliated cyanotic CHD,
- Completely repaired CHD with prosthetic material or device in the first 6 months after repair,
- Repaired CHD with residual defect near patch or device, or
- Valvulopathy developing after heart transplant.[40]

Transitions

Yet another critical aspect of caring for the adolescent with CHD is enabling a successful transition to adult providers. This process should ideally be initiated in early adolescence and completed by age 21 years. Although changes in insurance coverage and emotional attachment to a pediatric provider may create barriers, these are not insurmountable. Factors such as adolescents attending appointments without parents and the current primary care provider offering a recommendation for an adult provider can help facilitate these transitions.[41,42] In fact, ensuring the adult with CHD remains in a medical home and is not lost to follow-up may be one of the most valuable services a pediatric primary care provider can offer.

SUMMARY

Even children born with complex CHD and multiple extracardiac anomalies may survive to adulthood due to recent advances in the fields of pediatric cardiology and congenital heart surgery. Optimizing the growth, development, and quality of life for these children remains a challenge for primary care providers and pediatric subspecialists alike. Providers should continue to collaborate to meet the health care needs of this growing population. In addition, pediatric primary care providers and pediatric cardiologists should strive to prepare these children for a seamless transition to adulthood and adult care providers.

CLINICS CARE POINTS

- Consider discussion of any newly identified genetic abnormality in a child or child's first-degree relative with a geneticist or pediatric cardiologist if the cardiac implications are unclear.

- Recommend fetal echocardiogram screening to families when appropriate, as this screening has improved mortality in critical CHD.

- Do not assume that normal prenatal screening excludes CHD. This screening is not well standardized and still has limitations in detecting some forms of CHD.

- Do not assume that normal newborn pulse oximetry screening excludes CHD. Newborn hospitalization duration varies and the transition from fetal to postnatal circulation occurs at a variable rate.

- The timing of symptom emergence can help refine the list of potential diagnoses in children with suspected CHD.

- Have a low threshold to refer children with CHD for formal developmental assessment due to the increased risk of developmental delay.

- Carefully monitor growth in children with CHD, as the risk of obesity and obesity-related comorbidities is similar to the general population.

- Screen for psychiatric comorbidities in children and adolescents with CHD due to the increased risk of mental illness.

- Encourage children with CHD and repaired CHD to have regular dental care; however, only a limited number of these children require endocarditis prophylaxis based on current guidelines.

- Plan how and when to transition children with CHD to adult providers so they are not lost to follow-up.

DISCLOSURE

The authors have nothing to disclose.

REFERENCES

1. Collaborators GCHD. Global, regional, and national burden of congenital heart disease, 1990-2017: a systematic analysis for the Global Burden of Disease Study 2017. Lancet Child Adolesc Health 2020;4(3):185–200.

2. Burchill LJ, Gao L, Kovacs AH, et al. Hospitalization trends and health resource use for adult congenital heart disease-related heart failure. J Am Heart Assoc 2018;7(15):e008775.
3. Lantin-Hermoso MR, Berger S, Bhatt AB, et al. The care of children with congenital heart disease in their primary medical home. Pediatrics 2017;140(5): e20172607.
4. Pierpont ME, Brueckner M, Chung WK, et al. Genetic basis for congenital heart disease: revisited: a scientific statement from the American Heart Association. Circulation 2018;138(21):e653–711.
5. Online Mendelian Inheritance in Man, OMIM. Available at: https://omim.org. Accessed January 30, 2020.
6. Donofrio MT, Moon-Grady AJ, Hornberger LK, et al. Diagnosis and treatment of fetal cardiac disease: a scientific statement from the American Heart Association. Circulation 2014;129(21):2183–242.
7. Stoll C, Dott B, Alembik Y, et al. Associated noncardiac congenital anomalies among cases with congenital heart defects. Eur J Med Genet 2015;58(2):75–85.
8. Stümpflen I, Stümpflen A, Wimmer M, et al. Effect of detailed fetal echocardiography as part of routine prenatal ultrasonographic screening on detection of congenital heart disease. Lancet 1996;348(9031):854–7.
9. Yagel S, Weissman A, Rotstein Z, et al. Congenital heart defects: natural course and in utero development. Circulation 1997;96(2):550–5.
10. Pinto NM, Henry KA, Grobman WA, et al. Physician barriers and facilitators for screening for congenital heart disease with routine obstetric ultrasound: a national united states survey. J Ultrasound Med 2020;39(6):1143–53.
11. Holland BJ, Myers JA, Woods CR. Prenatal diagnosis of critical congenital heart disease reduces risk of death from cardiovascular compromise prior to planned neonatal cardiac surgery: a meta-analysis. Ultrasound Obstet Gynecol 2015; 45(6):631–8.
12. Quartermain MD, Pasquali SK, Hill KD, et al. Variation in prenatal diagnosis of congenital heart disease in infants. Pediatrics 2015;136(2):e378–85.
13. Brown J, Holland B. Successful fetal tele-echo at a small regional hospital. Telemed J E Health 2017;23(6):485–92. https://doi.org/10.1089/tmj.2016.0141.
14. Finnemore A, Groves A. Physiology of the fetal and transitional circulation. Semin Fetal Neonatal Med 2015;20(4):210–6.
15. Kliegman R, St. Geme J, Blum N, et al. Nelson textbook of pediatrics. 21st edition. Philadelphia, PA: Elsevier; 2020. p. 2.
16. Rios DR, Bhattacharya S, Levy PT, et al. Circulatory insufficiency and hypotension related to the ductus arteriosus in neonates. Front Pediatr 2018;6:62.
17. Kemper AR, Mahle WT, Martin GR, et al. Strategies for implementing screening for critical congenital heart disease. Pediatrics 2011;128(5):e1259–67.
18. Mahle WT, Newburger JW, Matherne GP, et al. Role of pulse oximetry in examining newborns for congenital heart disease: a scientific statement from the American Heart Association and American Academy of Pediatrics. Circulation 2009; 120(5):447–58.
19. Plana MN, Zamora J, Suresh G, et al. Pulse oximetry screening for critical congenital heart defects. Cochrane Database Syst Rev 2018;3:CD011912.
20. Mahle WT, Martin GR, Beekman RH, et al, Committee SoCaCSE. Endorsement of health and human services recommendation for pulse oximetry screening for critical congenital heart disease. Pediatrics 2012;129(1):190–2.
21. Files MD, Morray B. Total anomalous pulmonary venous connection: preoperative anatomy, physiology, imaging, and interventional management of postoperative

pulmonary venous obstruction. Semin Cardiothorac Vasc Anesth 2017;21(2): 123–31.

22. Kliegman R, St. Geme J, Blum N, et al. Nelson textbook of pediatrics. 21st edition. Philadelphia, PA: Elsevier; 2020. p. 13.

23. Puri K, Allen HD, Qureshi AM. Congenital heart disease. Pediatr Rev 2017;38(10): 471–86. https://doi.org/10.1542/pir.2017-0032.

24. Kliegman R, St. Geme J, Blum N, et al. Nelson textbook of pediatrics. 21st edition. Philadelphia, PA: Elsevier; 2020. p. 9.

25. Nguyen L, Cook SC. Coarctation of the aorta: strategies for improving outcomes. Cardiol Clin 2015;33(4):521–30, vii.

26. Dijkema EJ, Leiner T, Grotenhuis HB. Diagnosis, imaging and clinical management of aortic coarctation. Heart 2017;103(15):1148–55.

27. Kliegman R, St. Geme J, Blum N, et al. Nelson textbook of pediatrics. 21st edition. Philadelphia, PA: Elsevier; 2020. p. 12.

28. Villafañe J, Feinstein JA, Jenkins KJ, et al. Hot topics in tetralogy of Fallot. J Am Coll Cardiol 2013;62(23):2155–66.

29. Lannering K, Bartos M, Mellander M. Late diagnosis of coarctation despite prenatal ultrasound and postnatal pulse oximetry. Pediatrics 2015;136(2):e406–12.

30. Anderson RH, Cook AC. Morphology of the functionally univentricular heart. Cardiol Young 2004;14(Suppl 1):3–12.

31. Kliegman R, St. Geme J, Blum N, et al. Nelson textbook of pediatrics. 21st edition. Philadelphia, PA: Elsevier; 2020. p. 7.

32. Saito T, Ohta K, Nakayama Y, et al. Natural history of medium-sized atrial septal defect in pediatric cases. J Cardiol 2012;60(3):248–51.

33. Marino BS, Lipkin PH, Newburger JW, et al. Neurodevelopmental outcomes in children with congenital heart disease: evaluation and management: a scientific statement from the American Heart Association. Circulation 2012;126(9): 1143–72.

34. Ryan KR, Jones MB, Allen KY, et al. Neurodevelopmental outcomes among children with congenital heart disease: at-risk populations and modifiable risk factors. World J Pediatr Congenit Heart Surg 2019;10(6):750–8.

35. Daymont C, Neal A, Prosnitz A, et al. Growth in children with congenital heart disease. Pediatrics 2013;131(1):e236–42.

36. Pinto NM, Marino BS, Wernovsky G, et al. Obesity is a common comorbidity in children with congenital and acquired heart disease. Pediatrics 2007;120(5): e1157–64.

37. Calderon J, Bonnet D, Courtin C, et al. Executive function and theory of mind in school-aged children after neonatal corrective cardiac surgery for transposition of the great arteries. Research Support, Non-U.S. Gov't. Dev Med Child Neurol 2010;52(12):1139–44.

38. Khanna AD, Duca LM, Kay JD, et al. Prevalence of mental illness in adolescents and adults with congenital heart disease from the colorado congenital heart defect surveillance system. Am J Cardiol 2019;124(4):618–26.

39. DeMaso DR, Calderon J, Taylor GA, et al. Psychiatric disorders in adolescents with single ventricle congenital heart disease. Pediatrics 2017;139(3):e20162241.

40. Wilson W, Taubert KA, Gewitz M, et al. Prevention of infective endocarditis: guidelines from the American Heart Association: a guideline from the American Heart Association Rheumatic Fever, Endocarditis, and Kawasaki Disease Committee, Council on Cardiovascular Disease in the Young, and the Council on Clinical Cardiology, Council on Cardiovascular Surgery and Anesthesia, and the Quality of

Care and Outcomes Research Interdisciplinary Working Group. Circulation 2007; 116(15):1736–54.

41. Everitt IK, Gerardin JF, Rodriguez FH, et al. Improving the quality of transition and transfer of care in young adults with congenital heart disease. Congenit Heart Dis 2017;12(3):242–50.

42. Reid GJ, Irvine MJ, McCrindle BW, et al. Prevalence and correlates of successful transfer from pediatric to adult health care among a cohort of young adults with complex congenital heart defects. Pediatrics 2004;113(3 Pt 1):e197–205.

Pediatric Hypertension

Christopher Fox, MD, CAQ-SM[a,b,*]

KEYWORDS

- Hypertension • Pediatric hypertension • Elevated blood pressure
- Pediatric screening • Pediatric management

KEY POINTS

- The incidence rate of pediatric hypertension is between 2% and 4%; however, it is as high as 24% in obese children.
- There is strong evidence linking pediatric hypertension to cardiovascular disease in adults.
- Early recognition and intervention are key to prevent long-term complications.

INTRODUCTION
Epidemiology

Hypertension in the pediatric population has been an increasing concern over the last decade. Recent epidemiologic studies have shown an incidence rate in children and adolescents from 0.8% to as high as 4% and up to 24% in obese children.[1–3] The national average for obesity in the pediatric population is 35%, which has quadrupled in the last 40 years.[2,4] Rates of pediatric hypertension show an increasing linear relationship to increasing adiposity.[2] Boys have consistently shown a higher prevalence than girls.[2,5] There is also a higher prevalence among Hispanic and non-Hispanic African Americans.[2,5] Children classified as obese (body mass index [BMI] 95% to 98%) had a twofold increase in hypertension compared with healthy weight children, and severely obese (BMI >99%) have a fourfold increase..[3]

The American Heart Association (AHA) and the American Academy of Pediatrics (AAP) recently updated guidelines for diagnosing pediatric hypertension. The national prevalence has consistently been around 2% to 4%; however, with the recent change, the incidence of diagnosing prehypertension has increased.[1] A study by Bell and colleagues in the Houston area found a 1.5% increase in the prevalence of elevated blood pressure or previously labeled prehypertension in their study population by reclassifying to the new AAP criteria.[1]

[a] University of Missouri-Kansas City, School of Medicine, Kansas City, MO, USA; [b] Department of Community and Family Medicine, Truman Medical Centers, Kansas City, MO, USA
* 600 NE Adams Dairy Pkwy, Blue Springs, MO 64014, USA.
E-mail addresses: chrisfox.m@gmail.com; Christopher.fox@tmcmed.org

Prim Care Clin Office Pract 48 (2021) 367–378
https://doi.org/10.1016/j.pop.2021.04.001
0095-4543/21/© 2021 Elsevier Inc. All rights reserved.

There have been numerous studies that show that elevated blood pressure in childhood increases the risk for adult hypertension and other comorbidities.[2,6] This highlights the importance of making an early diagnosis but also in identifying the steps for early intervention.

Definitions

The definition of pediatric hypertension was recently updated by the AAP in 2017. Previously the Fourth Report (2004) defined normal blood pressure as systolic (SBP) and diastolic blood pressure (DBP) reading less than 90 percentile based on age, sex, and height normograms. Prehypertension was defined as blood pressure greater than 120/90 (or 90th) to 95th percentile. Hypertension was defined as SBP and/or DBP greater than the 95th percentile.[7,8]

The AAP updated these definitions as follows: for children over 13 years of age, the definition for hypertension remains the same as the 2017 AHA adult classification.[2,7,9] The term prehypertension has also been reclassified as elevated blood pressure. The definitions of elevated blood pressure under the age of 13 years remains SBP and/or DBP in the 90th to 94th percentiles. Stage 1 hypertension is defined as blood pressure readings in the 95th to 99th percentiles, and stage 2 hypertension is defined as blood pressure readings greater than the 95th percentile plus 12 mm Hg.

The AAP has developed tables based on normative data of blood pressure in healthy children. These tables factor in the child's height, age, and sex and allow comparison of blood pressure readings to these normative classifications in order to determine if a child's blood pressure is elevated. The normative tables were also updated, which removed the values of children who were overweight or obese (BMI >85th percentile).[2] Studies looking at these updated normograms have shown remarkably high sensitivities of 99.9%; however, specificity was around 84%.[10] The rates of hypertension have remained steady; however, there has been an increase in the diagnosis of elevated blood pressure as previously discussed.[1] These normative tables can be found on the AAP's Web site for clinical use.

https://pediatrics.aappublications.org/content/140/3/e20171904/tab-figures-data.

Screening Recommendations

Currently the AAP recommends that all children be screened for hypertension starting at the age of 3 years, and this should be continued yearly (Grade C recommendation). If the child has obesity, renal disease, coarctation of the aorta, diabetes, or is on a medication that can increase blood pressure, then it is recommended that he or she has his or her blood pressure measured at every health care encounter (Grade C recommendation). Children under the age of 3 years who have medical conditions making them higher risk for hypertension such as prematurity, low birth weight, kidney dysmorphia, or a maternal history of smoking should also have the blood pressure monitored at their routine wellness visits.[2] The latest United States Preventive Services Task Force (USPSTF) update from 2020 determined there was insufficient evidence to recommend screening for primary hypertension in asymptomatic children and adolescents.[11-14]

ETIOLOGY AND RISK FACTORS FOR DEVELOPMENT
Primary versus Secondary

Pediatric hypertension can further be classified as either primary (essential) hypertension or secondary hypertension. Secondary hypertension is hypertension that develops secondary to another identifiable cause. Primary hypertension that does not have an identifiable secondary cause is therefore a diagnosis of exclusion.

There are some identified risk factors for the development of primary pediatric hypertension. A family history of hypertension or cardiovascular disease is a known risk factor for the development of hypertension, especially in older children.[15] Male gender, Hispanic decent, and African American decent are also known risk factors for the development of primary hypertension.[2,16–18] This is suggestive of a genetic basis for the development of primary hypertension that is, poorly understood.[2,15–17]

Overweight and obese children also have an increased risk of developing primary hypertension as discussed in the introduction. Insulin resistance and sleep disorders are both chronic conditions that have independently shown an increased risk for the development of hypertension. Sleep disorders that are associated with pediatric hypertension include obstructive sleep apnea, snoring, and fragmented sleep.[16,18] Chronic kidney disease, low birth weight, or a maternal history of smoking are also additional risk factors.[18] Studies show breastfeeding has a protective relationship with hypertension and may be linked to lower systolic pressures later in life.[16,18,19] There have also been several studies looking at the correlation between uric acid levels and the development of pediatric hypertension. Studies have shown a positive relationship between uric acid levels greater than 5.5 mg/dL and elevated blood pressure in adolescents.[16,20] (**Box 1**).

Secondary hypertension can be caused by several different underlying medical pathologies that need to be excluded prior to the diagnosis of primary hypertension (**Table 1**).

EVALUATION
Blood Pressure Measurement

Any child over the age of 3 years with obesity or other risk factors known to predispose them to the development of hypertension should have their blood pressure measured at every health care encounter.[2] It is also recommended to have multiple readings during the same visit and across additional office visits to evaluate children whose blood pressure is reading elevated. There is a wide degree of variability in pediatric blood pressure readings, and outside influences such as stress and anxiety can cause those blood pressure readings to be momentarily elevated.[2]

Box 1
Risk factors for the development of primary hypertension in children and adolescents

1. Family history of hypertension or cardiovascular disease
2. Male gender
3. Hispanic decent
4. African American decent
5. Overweight/obesity
6. Insulin resistance
7. Sleep disorders
8. Low birth weight
9. Maternal history of smoking
10. Chronic kidney disease
11. Elevated uric acid levels

Table 1
Etiologies of secondary hypertension in children

Etiology	History	Physical Examination	Diagnostic Tests
Coarctation of the aorta	Family history	Diminished femoral pulses, Difference in blood pressure between right and left arms	Echocardiogram
Cushing syndrome	Family history	Acne, hirsutism, obesity, moon facies	Cortisol levels
Renal artery stenosis	History of umbilical catheterization	None	Renin, aldosterone, renal Doppler
Drug-induced	Medication history, illicit drug use	Tachycardia Diaphoresis	Urine drug screen
Hyperthyroidism	Family history, weight loss, diaphoresis	Tachycardia, exophthalmos, thyromegaly	Thyroid function tests
Congenital adrenal hyperplasia	Family history	Ambiguous genitalia	Aldosterone, renin, hypokalemia
Obstructive sleep apnea	Snoring, obesity	Mallampati score, tonsillar hypertrophy	Sleep study
Pheochromocytoma	Flushing, sweating, tremors, palpitations	Diaphoresis, tachycardia, pallor	Plasma and urine catecholamines
Renal parenchymal disease	Family history, enuresis	Hematuria, edema	Blood urea nitrogen, creatinine, urinalysis, renal ultrasound
Autoimmune disease	Family history Joint pain, fevers, weight loss	Synovitis, hematuria, mallor rash	Complete blood cell count, basic metabolic panel, inflammatory markers, autoimmune laboratory testing

Data from Refs.[2,18,31]

The child's blood pressure can be measured by either using an oscillometric automated device or by an auscultatory method.[2] When measuring a child's blood pressure, selection of the appropriate cuff is critical. If a cuff that is too large or too small for the child's arm is used, it will not yield an accurate reading. The current recommendations by the AAP are to use the midarm circumference to determine the appropriate cuff size. This location is the midpoint between the acromion of the scapula and the olecranon of the elbow.

After measurement of the child's blood pressure, the pressure should be compared with the normograms discussed in the definitions section. If the blood pressure is above the 90th percentile for that child, then a minimum of 2 more measurements should be taken at that office visit and the average of all 3 measurements determined. This should then be the blood pressure used to determine the child's blood pressure category[2] (**Fig. 1**).

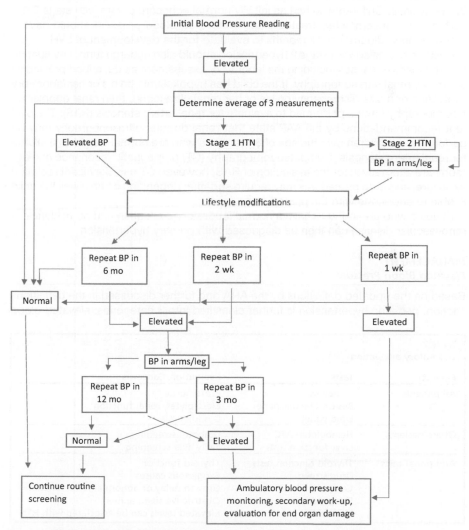

Fig. 1. Pediatric hypertension evaluation.

Primary versus Secondary

After the determination of the child's blood pressure category, the child may require additional work-up to determine the etiology of his or her hypertension. Children found to be in stage 2 hypertension are at higher risk for having secondary hypertension. These children should undergo further laboratory evaluation to rule out renal or endocrine causes of their hypertension (**Table 2**).

A diagnosis of stage 2 hypertension also warrants further evaluation to rule out of end organ damage. Echocardiography was determined by the Fourth Report to be the recommended tool for evaluation of left ventricular hypertrophy (LVH) associated with pediatric hypertension. Studies have shown an independent relationship of LVH to adverse cardiac outcomes as an adult.[2] The AAP currently recommends an echocardiogram be performed on children in consideration for pharmacologic management of hypertension. Children found to have LVH on their initial echocardiogram should have a repeat echocardiogram in 6 to 12 months to evaluate for progression of the disease. Children who had an initially normal echocardiogram with stage 2 hypertension or incompletely treated stage 1/elevated blood pressure should have a repeat echocardiogram at 12 months to evaluate for the development of LVH.

Children classified with stage 2 hypertension should also undergo further evaluation for renovascular causes including the laboratory assessment as described previously as well as renal ultrasonography. If the child has hypokalemia on his or her laboratory evaluation or a size discrepancy on his or her renal ultrasound, then renal doppler ultrasonography can be performed to evaluate for renal artery stenosis (RAS). The current recommendations by the AAP state that renal doppler ultrasonography may be performed on children over the age of 8 years and who are normal weight to evaluate for renal artery stenosis. Computed tomography (CT) or magnetic resonance angiography are alternatives for the evaluation of RAS; however, CT has significant radiation exposure, and both procedures may require sedation depending on how well the child is able to cooperate with the procedure.[2]

Patients who are found to have a normal laboratory evaluation and no evidence of renovascular disease can then be diagnosed with primary hypertension.

MANAGEMENT
Elevated Blood Pressure

Based on the updated definitions by the AHA and further discussed in the definitions section, pediatric hypertension is further classified into 3 categories: elevated blood

Table 2
Laboratory evaluation

Patients	Tests	Evaluation/Concerns
All patients	Urinalysis	Proteinuria
	Basic metabolic panel	Electrolytes, renal function
	Lipid panel	Dyslipidemia
Obese patients	Hemoglobin A1C	Diabetes screening
	Liver function tests	Fatty liver screening
Additional tests	Thyroid function tests	Thyroid function
	Drug screen	Exogenous causes
	Complete blood count	Growth delay or abnormal renal function
	Sleep study	Obstructive sleep apnea
	Uric acid	Elevated levels can be associated with HTN

Data from Refs.[2,16]

pressure (formerly prehypertension), stage 1 hypertension, and stage 2 hypertension.[2,21] If a child's blood pressure falls into the elevated blood pressure category during his or her routine screening, the blood pressure should be measured again during the visit. If it then normalizes, the child can continue routine follow-ups with yearly blood pressure screening (see **Fig. 1**).

Children whose blood pressure remains greater than the 90% percentile but less than the 95% percentile on repeat measurement are considered to have elevated blood pressure. The first recommended intervention is lifestyle modifications. These can include:

- Decreasing dietary sodium
- Healthier eating habits
- Weight loss
- Nutrition management or consultation with a registered dietician
- Encouragement of physical activity (guidelines can be discussed)
- Promotion of healthy sleep patterns

These children should have their blood pressure measured again in 6 months by auscultation.[2] If their blood pressure remains elevated at 6 months, then repeating the measurement in both arms and a lower extremity is recommended to evaluate for aortic coarctation. Lifestyle changes and weight management should be discussed again, and referrals may be warranted. The child should then be followed again in 6 months. If blood pressure remains elevated after 12 months, ambulatory blood pressure monitoring and further work-up should be considered to rule out secondary causes. In children whose blood pressure continues to fail to normalize after conservative management, pharmacologic management can be considered and is discussed further in the stage 2 hypertension management section (see **Fig. 1**).

Stage 1 Hypertension

Stage 1 hypertension is diagnosed when a child's (<13 year old) blood pressure remains over the 95% percentile but less than the 99% percentile. For an adolescent (>13 year old), this is defined as a blood pressure between 130/80 and 139/89.

A diagnosis of stage 1 hypertension in an asymptomatic child can initially be treated with lifestyle changes, conservative management, and close monitoring/follow-up. It is currently recommended that any child initially diagnosed with stage 1 hypertension be followed in 1 to 2 weeks and have his or her blood pressure rechecked by auscultation.[2]

Recheck blood pressure in both arms and a lower extremity if elevated readings persist. Should there be difficulty implementing lifestyle changes, then a nutrition consultation may be warranted with follow-up in 3 months.

Initiate ambulatory blood pressure monitoring and pharmacologic treatment if the child's blood pressure remains elevated after 3 visits. Subspecialty referral can be considered to nephrology or cardiology for the child with persistently elevated blood pressures.

Stage 2 Hypertension

Stage 2 hypertension is defined as a blood pressure greater than the 95% + 12 mm Hg or greater than 140/90, whichever is lower.

For a child or adolescent diagnosed with stage 2 hypertension, it is recommended that the blood pressure measurement be repeated in both upper and a lower extremity at that visit. The child should be referred to nutrition or weight management.

Follow-up measurements of blood pressure should occur within 1 week. If the child remains in the stage 2 hypertension category at follow-up, then ambulatory blood pressure monitoring should be performed, further laboratory and imaging evaluations ordered, and pharmacologic treatment initiated.2,21 A subspecialty referral can be considered in patients with both stage 1 and stage 2 hypertension.

Any child who presents with stage 1 or 2 hypertension and is symptomatic should be referred to the emergency room for acute blood pressure management. These symptoms could include seizures, lethargy, vision changes, altered mental status, headache, nausea, pulmonary edema, or other symptoms of congestive heart failure.[9] A study by Hamby and colleagues demonstrated that, on average, years passed prior to a child being referred to a nephrologist for hypertension despite remaining elevated at multiple visits.[22] It is important for clinicians to recognize these elevated blood pressures in order to make a timely diagnosis and referral if needed (see **Fig. 1**).

Pharmacologic Management

When considering starting a child diagnosed with primary hypertension on an anti-hypertensive medication much thought and discussion should go into the decision. Lifestyle modifications should fully be maximized prior to consideration of initiating pharmacologic therapy. However, if a child's blood pressure is staying in the stage 2 category, he or she has LVH on echocardiography, or he or she is symptomatic, then a pharmacologic agent should be initiated. For children started on pharmacologic management, follow-up every 4 to 6 weeks is recommended initially for dose titration and then every 3 to 6 months for monitoring.[21]

Anti-hypertensives have been less studied in children; therefore less is known about the long-term outcomes of these medications compared with adults. Many of these medications are considered off-label use in the pediatric population.[23] Initial treatment is recommended with an angiotensin-converting enzyme (ACE) inhibitor or angiotensin receptor blocker (ARB), long-acting calcium channel blocker, or thiazide diuretic. Beta blockers are not recommended as initial agents.[2] In adolescents, careful attention needs to be paid to a sexual history in girls, as ACE inhibitors and ARBs are contra-indicated during pregnancy. In children with hypertension and chronic kidney disease, proteinuria, or diabetes, an ACE inhibitor or ARB is recommended as first-line treatment.[2]

There has also been an association found between elevated uric acid levels and primary hypertension. Treatment of these uric acid levels with a uric acid-lowering agent may help in reducing blood pressure; however, more studies are needed to clarify the utility.[2,16,23]

DISCUSSION
Long-Term Complications

The development of hypertension in a child can have long-term implications, especially if elevated blood pressures persist. Persistently elevated blood pressures can damage the small vessels, creating target organ damage including involvement of the eyes, kidneys, heart, brain, and arteries in children.[10] There have also been studies showing a correlation between pediatric hypertension and the development of cardiovascular disease as an adult.[2] Epidemiologic studies have shown that elevated blood pressures in children as young as age 12 may increase the incidence of adult cardiovascular disease.[24]

LVH is a known complication of pediatric hypertension. This occurs as the left ventricular mass is increased in response to elevated blood pressures. A study by Conkar and colleagues of 82 children with pediatric hypertension showed rates of target organ damage including retinopathy (35%), microalbuminuria (26%), and increased left ventricular mass (17%).[24] LVH is a known surrogate marker for morbidity and mortality associated with pediatric hypertension.[10] The prevalence of LVH in children and adolescents has been difficult to determine given the multiple definitions that are used. In essential hypertension, severe LVH with left ventricular mass index (LVMI) above 51g has been estimated to be 10% to 15%.[10] The presence of LVH in children with hypertension should prompt treatment with the goal of LVH reversal. Hypertension remains a rare cause of heart failure in children.[10]

The development of chronic kidney disease is another potential long-term complication of persistent uncontrolled hypertension in children. Microalbuminuria is a marker of potential development of hypertensive kidney injury in children, and a positive test should prompt pharmacologic treatment.[2,16] Treatment in adults with an ACE inhibitor or ARB has been shown to effectively reduce microalbuminuria, and improvement in microalbuminuria has been associated with reduced cardiovascular risk; however, these studies have not been successfully reproduced in a pediatric population.[2,10]

Damage to the microvasculature affecting the retina is another known complication of pediatric hypertension.[16] The rates of retinopathy associated with pediatric hypertension have been estimated as high as 8% to 35%.[24,25] A formal retinal examination should be considered for children diagnosed with hypertension, especially stage 2 hypertension. There has also been evidence of impaired cognition in children diagnosed with hypertension and documented improvement with treatment.[16,26]

Many of these long-term complications do lead to permanent organ damage and morbidity and mortality as an adult; however, it has also been demonstrated that if hypertension is controlled some of the target organ damage may be reversible.

Prevention

The incidence of primary hypertension in pediatrics has closely mirrored the increasing rates of obesity in the pediatric population. Currently around one-third of children in the Unites States are affected by overweight or obesity, and the rates increase with age.[27] When discussing prevention of pediatric hypertension, the discussion of pediatric obesity must be at the center.

Physical activity is a key component to the prevention of pediatric obesity and hypertension and one of the first recommended lifestyle modifications for those diagnosed with elevated blood pressure or hypertension. Currently the CDC recommend a goal of 60 minutes of moderate-to-vigorous physical activity daily for children ages 6 to 17 years; however, only about 33% are achieving this goal.[2,16,28] The recommendations for children under 6 year old is to be active throughout the day. Adults should help find activities to keep children active and encourage the children to remain engaged in these activities.[29]

Nutrition management and sleep hygiene are also key components to prevention and lifestyle modifications. There have been studies showing evidence of an association between shortened sleep duration and childhood obesity.[27] A detailed sleep history and input from parents can help identify poor sleep patterns. A sleep study can also be considered for a child with a history of snoring.

Sports Clearance/Preparticipation Examinations

All athletes participating in organized sports are required to undergo a preparticipation exam (PPE) to determine if they can safely participate in sport. The overarching goal of the PPE is to promote an environment of safety in athletics and provide a screening opportunity for injuries and underlying medical conditions that could predispose the athlete to an adverse outcome.[30]

Hypertension is one of the most commonly encountered pathologies at the PPE, and screening for hypertension is recommended for every PPE.[30] According to the PPE Monograph in association with the AAP, children with severe or stage 2 hypertension should not be initially cleared and undergo further work-up or specialty consultation. These athletes should avoid heavy intensity static exercises such as powerlifting and bodybuilding. Once the investigation is complete and blood pressure is controlled, then participation should be re-evaluated. Those with stage 1 hypertension or elevated blood pressure may be cleared for participation with the condition that the child follow-up for further evaluation of his or her elevated blood pressure.[30] Determining and ensuring parent and child understanding of the need for further work-up and any restrictions placed on the athlete are important. Discussing provisional clearance can be important to help with parent and athlete compliance. If an athlete fails to follow-up or complete the requested work-up, removal of the provisional clearance may be needed to ensure the continued safety of that athlete.

CLINICS CARE POINTS

- The incidence of pediatric hypertension is increasing in a linear relationship to the increasing rates of childhood obesity.
- Blood pressure should be measured at every well child examination starting at the age of 3 years and at every office visit for children who are at higher risk.
- Practitioners need to be aware of the pediatric normograms for comparison of blood pressures in the office and to assist in early diagnosis of pediatric hypertension.
- Multiple measurements of blood pressure should be made during an office visit if a child has an elevated blood pressure and the average used to determine blood pressure classification.
- Lifestyle modifications are first-line management for all asymptomatic patients; however, secondary causes and end organ damage need to be excluded in patients with stage 2 hypertension or persistently elevated blood pressure despite lifestyle modifications.
- Children with symptomatic hypertension should be evaluated in the emergency room for more prompt evaluation and management.

DISCLOSURE

The author has nothing to disclose.

REFERENCES

1. Bell CS, Samuel JP, Samuels JA. Prevalence of hypertension in children. Hypertension 2019;73(1):148–52.
2. Flynn JT, Kaelber DC, Baker-Smith CM, et al. Clinical practice guideline for screening and management of high blood pressure in children and adolescents. Pediatrics 2017;140(3). https://doi.org/10.1542/peds.2017-1904.
3. Parker ED, Sinaiko AR, Kharbanda EO, et al. Change in weight status and development of hypertension. Pediatrics 2016;137(3):e20151662.
4. Fryer C. Products - health E stats - prevalence of overweight and obesity among children and adolescents aged 2–19 years: United States, 1963–1965 through 2013–2014. 2016. Available at: https://www.cdc.gov/nchs/data/hestat/obesity_child_13_14/obesity_child_13_14.html. Accessed September 29, 2020.

5. Kit BK, Kuklina E, Carroll MD, et al. Prevalence of and trends in dyslipidemia and blood pressure among US children and adolescents, 1999-2012. JAMA Pediatr 2015;169(3):272–9.

6. Bucher BS, Ferrarini A, Weber N, et al. Primary hypertension in childhood. Curr Hypertens Rep 2013;15(5):444–52.

7. Genovesi S, Parati G, Giussani M, et al. How to apply European and American guidelines on high blood pressure in children and adolescents. A position paper endorsed by the Italian Society of Hypertension and the Italian Society of Pediatrics. High Blood Press Cardiovasc Prev 2020. https://doi.org/10.1007/s40292-020-00369-y [Review].

8. National High Blood Pressure Education Program Working Group on High Blood Pressure in Children and Adolescents. The fourth report on the diagnosis, evaluation, and treatment of high blood pressure in children and adolescents. Pediatrics 2004;114(2 Suppl 4th Report):555–76.

9. Baracco R. A practical guide to the management of severe hypertension in children. Paediatr Drugs 2020;22(1):13–20.

10. Zhang Y, Yang L, Hou Y, et al. Performance of the simplified American Academy of Pediatrics table to screen elevated blood pressure in children. JAMA Pediatr 2018;172(12):1196–8.

11. Moyer V. Screening for primary hypertension in children and adolescents: U.S Preventive Services Task Force recommendation statement. Pediatrics 2013; 132(5):907–14.

12. Unites States Preventative Services Task Force. High blood pressure in children and adolescents: screening. Available at: https://www.uspreventiveservic estaskforce.org/uspstf/recommendation/blood-pressure-in-children-and-adolesc ents-hypertension-screening#fullrecommendationstart. Accessed December 15, 2020.

13. Whelton PK, Carey RM, Aronow WS, et al. 2017 ACC/AHA/AAPA/ABC/ACPM/AGS/APhA/ASH/ASPC/NMA/PCNA guideline for the prevention, detection, evaluation, and management of high blood pressure in adults: a report of the American College of Cardiology/American Heart Association Task Force on Clinical Practice Guidelines. Circulation 2018;138(17):e484–594.

14. Woroniecki RP, Kahnauth A, Panesar LE, et al. Left ventricular hypertrophy in pediatric hypertension: a mini review. Front Pediatr 2017;5:101.

15. Matossian D. Pediatric Hypertension. Pediatr Ann 2018;47(12):e499–503.

16. Ahern D, Dixon E. Pediatric hypertension: a growing problem. Prim Care 2015; 42(1):143–50.

17. Guzman-Limon M, Samuels J. Pediatric hypertension: diagnosis, evaluation, and treatment. Pediatr Clin North Am 2019;66(1):45–57 [Review].

18. Riley M, Hernandez AK, Kuznia AL. High blood pressure in children and adolescents. Am Fam Physician 2018;98(8):486–94.

19. Owen CG, Whincup PH, Gilg JA, et al. Effect of breast feeding in infancy on blood pressure in later life: systematic review and meta-analysis. BMJ 2003;327(7425): 1189–95.

20. Raj M. Essential hypertension in adolescents and children: Recent advances in causative mechanisms. Indian J Endocrinol Metab 2011;15(Suppl 4):S367–73.

21. Sinha R, Saha A, Samuels J. American Academy of Pediatrics clinical practice guidelines for screening and management of high blood pressure in children and adolescents: what is new? Indian Pediatr 2019;56(4):317–21.

22. Hamby T, Pueringer MR, Noorani S, et al. Time to referral to a nephrology clinic for pediatric hypertension. Pediatr Nephrol 2020;35(5):907–10.

23. Misurac J, Nichols KR, Wilson AC. Pharmacologic management of pediatric hypertension. Paediatr Drugs 2016;18(1):31–43.
24. Conkar S, Yılmaz E, Hacıkara Ş, et al. Is daytime systolic load an important risk factor for target organ damage in pediatric hypertension? J Clin Hypertens (Greenwich) 2015;17(10):760–6.
25. Foster BJ, Ali H, Mamber S, et al. Prevalence and severity of hypertensive retinopathy in children. Clin Pediatr (Phila) 2009;48(9):926–30.
26. Taylor-Zapata P, Baker-Smith CM, Burckart G, et al. Research gaps in primary pediatric hypertension. Pediatrics 2019;143(5). https://doi.org/10.1542/peds.2018-3517.
27. Kumar S, Kelly AS. Review of childhood obesity: from epidemiology, etiology, and comorbidities to clinical assessment and treatment. Mayo Clin Proc 2017;92(2):251–65.
28. Foster C, Moore JB, Singletary CR, et al. Physical activity and family-based obesity treatment: a review of expert recommendations on physical activity in youth. Clin Obes 2018;8(1):68–79.
29. Centers for Disease Control and Prevention. Youth physical activity guidelines. Centers for Disease Control and Prevention; 2019. Available at: www.cdc.gov/healthyschools/physicalactivity/guidelines.htm.
30. Bernhardt DT, Roberts WO. PPE: preparticipation physical evaluation. Itasca (IL): American Academy of Pediatrics; 2019.
31. Saida K, Kamei K, Hamada R, et al. A simple refined approach for renovascular hypertension in children: a ten-year experience. Pediatr Int 2020.

Pediatric Asthma for the Primary Care Physician

Kevin W. Gray, MD, CAQ-SM

KEYWORDS

- Pediatric • Asthma • Wheezing

KEY POINTS

- Asthma is the most common chronic illness in children and a common cause of morbidity within the pediatric population.
- Asthma is characterized by fluctuating expiratory airflow limitation.
- Diagnosis should be made at the time of initial presentation with objective spirometry or peak expiratory flow testing.
- The extent of expiratory limitation will guide the stepwise approach to treatment.
- New research has changed treatment algorithms.

INTRODUCTION

Asthma is a Greek word derived from *aazein*, a verb meaning to exhale with an open mouth. Historically, any patient with shortness of breath was asthmatic. It was not until the nineteenth century that asthma was used to describe the disease process described in current times. It was at this time that the disease was clarified as "Paroxysmal dyspnoea of a peculiar character with intervals of healthy respiration between attacks."[1]

Asthma is the most common chronic disease in children, which is usually characterized by chronic inflammation of the airways of the lungs.[2] Common symptoms include wheezing, shortness of breath, cough, and chest tightness.[3] These symptoms are often variable and present with variable airflow limitation.[4]

Airway hyperreactivity and inflammation are associated with asthma, although they are not necessary for diagnosis. Airflow limitation is typically expiratory in nature, while also being variable. Triggers that can precipitate exacerbation and worsen disease control include exercise, allergens, airway irritants, viral infections, and weather changes.

Department of Community and Family Medicine, Truman Medical Center–Lakewood, 7900 Lee's Summit Road, Kansas City, MO 64139, USA
E-mail address: Kevin.Gray@tmcmed.org

Prim Care Clin Office Pract 48 (2021) 379–394
https://doi.org/10.1016/j.pop.2021.04.007
0095-4543/21/© 2021 Elsevier Inc. All rights reserved.
primarycare.theclinics.com

PATHOPHYSIOLOGY

Asthma is a heterogenous disease with complex pathophysiology. Leading the pathophysiology is airway hyperreactivity. An exaggerated bronchoconstrictor response is implicated, usually in the presence of different stimuli. Atopy with increase in immunoglobulin E (IgE) level and response of type IV hypersensitivity are implicated in exacerbation of disease.[5,6]

Asthma symptoms are caused at a basic level by airway narrowing. This variable airflow limitation occurs by several proposed mechanisms. First, bronchial smooth muscle contraction decreases airway size and is targeted by bronchodilator therapy. Airway edema by inflammatory mediated microvascular leakage causes additional narrowing. Mucosal thickening and fibroblast mediated remodeling may occur with severe disease and is not reversed with current treatments. Mucus plugging is the result of excess secretion of mucus, leading to occlusion of the small airways.[6]

EPIDEMIOLOGY

- Worldwide, chronic asthma in children affects more than 300 million individuals with prevalence increasing among pediatric populations.[1,4]
- Asthma is the leading chronic disease in children.
- In the United States, more than 5.5 million children are affected, with 7.5% of children currently have a diagnosis of asthma.
- Yearly costs exceed 56 billion dollars.
- Asthma is the third most common cause of hospitalization of children under 15 years of age.
- A primary diagnosis of asthma results in 1.6 million Emergency Department (ED) visits each year.
- Asthma accounts for more than 10.5 million missed school days per year.
- Asthma accounts for 9.8 million physician office visits.
- Boys are affected more often than girls in the pediatric population.
- The death rate is higher in African Americans than other ethnicities.

DIAGNOSIS

Correctly diagnosing asthma is important and is ideally completed before initiating treatment. The diagnosis becomes difficult to confirm once patients are started on controller treatments. Early diagnosis is important to avoid unnecessary treatment or overtreatment, and for prompt evaluation of other important diagnoses.[5]

HISTORY

Childhood symptoms and personal or family history of atopic disease (allergic rhinitis, atopic dermatitis, asthma) should be elucidated on initial history taking. Although these are not specific for asthma and are absent in some asthma phenotypes, it is important to note these, as they increase the probability that symptoms are related to asthma.[5]

Features increasing likelihood of asthma:

- Presence of more than one of the following symptoms: wheeze, cough, shortness of breath, cough, chest tightness
- Respiratory symptoms worse at night or in early morning
- Symptoms that vary in intensity and over time

- Symptoms triggered by viral infections, exercise, allergens, weather changes, laughter, irritants

Features decreasing likelihood of asthma:

- Isolated cough without other respiratory symptoms
- Chronic sputum production
- Shortness of breath with dizziness, light-headedness, or paresthesia
- Exercise-induced dyspnea with noisy inspiration

Differential diagnosis:

Age 6 to 11:
    Chronic upper airway cough syndrome (postnasal drip)
    Inhaled foreign body
    Bronchiectasis
    Primary ciliary dyskinesia
    Congenital heart disease
    Bronchopulmonary dysplasia
    Cystic fibrosis
    Tuberculosis
    Gastroesophageal reflux
Age 12+:
    Inducible laryngeal obstruction (vocal cord dysfunction)
    Chronic sinusitis
    Hyperventilation
    Dysfunctional breathing
    Alpha1-antitrypsin deficiency

Increasing interest has been devoted to genetic components related to risk of asthma as well as to response to treatment. Many genes have been explored with a focus on increased atopy, airway hyperreactivity, and inflammatory cytokine expression, and T-helper 1 and 2 concentrations have remained the focus of these explorations. HLA-DQB1 gene variant has shown increasing concentrations of IgE antibodies and atopy. In addition, several genes affecting the inflammatory cascade have been found to factor into the pathophysiology of airway hyperreactivity. Mutations in genes responsible for mucin production have been found to have greater prevalence in more severe asthma.[7–9]

Sex differences have also been implicated in asthma. In the pediatric population, asthma is almost twice as common in boys compared with girls. Although the exact reasoning is not clear, pediatric boys have smaller airways and lungs at younger ages.[10]

Asthma risk is also associated with various birth, and findings in infancy increase the risk of asthma in childhood. Early gestation, low birth weight, and higher weight gain early in life have all been found to increase this risk. In addition, children delivered by cesarean section have an increased risk of childhood asthma. This is thought to be due to differences seen in the normal microbiome, which seem to have a protective effect on development of atopic disease.[11]

Obesity in childhood is also found to be an independent risk factor for the development of childhood asthma. Alterations in airway functions, inflammatory predisposition, and increases in airway obstruction may explain this association. Paired with this, maternal prenatal obesity increases risk of childhood asthma and wheezing.[12]

Environmental allergen exposures are also well documented to increase symptoms, consistent with asthma early in life as well as the risk of childhood asthma. These include dust mites, cat dander, dog dander, Aspergillus, and cockroaches. Ingested allergen sensitization in childhood, including peanuts and tree nuts, is also a risk factor for asthma; however, antenatal exposure has not been shown to increase the risk in childhood. Although rhinitis does increase risk for asthma and allergen immunotherapy may decrease short-term asthma risk, this treatment has not been reliably shown to decrease long-term asthma risk.[13,14]

Infection with respiratory syncytial virus (RSV), rhinovirus, and parainfluenza virus causes bronchiolitis, which has significant symptom overlap with asthma. Rhinovirus infections in early childhood increase the risk of childhood asthma. In children hospitalized with RSV, around 40% experience either recurrent wheezing or childhood asthma. Unfortunately, neither RSV vaccination nor RSV monoclonal antibody therapy has been shown to reduce the risk of recurrent wheezing of early childhood or childhood asthma.[15]

Tobacco smoke exposure is commonly recognized as an exposure that is detrimental to respiratory health. Maternal smoking alters the development of fetal lung tissue. In children born to mothers who smoke during pregnancy, the risk or early childhood wheezing in the first year of life. Secondhand smoke exposure after birth similarly increases this risk in both infancy and childhood. In children with asthma, tobacco smoking worsens lung function, is associated with poor disease control, and renders chronic and acute exacerbation therapies less effective. Early data on vaping suggest negative effects on asthma symptoms.[16]

Air pollution is detrimental to respiratory health with both outdoor and indoor pollutants increasing childhood asthma risk. Children with homes and schools with high surrounding traffic density show increased risk of developing asthma. Children with prenatal exposure to outdoor pollutants are also affected. Indoor pollutants, such as exhaust and fumes of gas, and biomass fuels in addition to mold and cockroach infestations as mentioned earlier increase morbidity and deleteriously affect lung function.[17,18]

The study of maternal diet has not shown foods increase the risk of wheezing or asthma; however, antenatal ingestion of milk and peanuts, common allergenic foods, reduces the risk of allergy and asthma in children. Infants fed intact cow-milk or soy-based formula have a higher risk of wheezing in childhood when compared with breastfed children. The antenatal Western diet, which is generally high in processed foods and omega-6 fatty acids, is associated with increased risk of allergy and asthma. In high-risk individuals, antenatal supplementation with high-dose omega-3 fatty acids may decrease wheezing and asthma among preschool-aged children. A diet higher in omega-3 polyunsaturated fatty acids and lower in omega-6 fatty acids is associated with improved asthma control in school-aged children.[19]

Low vitamin D levels during pregnancy increase the risk of allergy and asthma. It is not clear if supplementation during pregnancy mitigates this risk. Inflammatory properties of both obesity and asthma have led to research about potential benefit of supplementation with the goal of exacerbation prevention. Studies are currently being conducted.[20–22]

Factors that may increase asthma risk:

- Genetics
- Early gestation
- Low birth weight
- Rapid early weight gain
- Cesarean section delivery
- Obesity

- Environmental and ingested allergens
- Infections (RSV, rhinovirus)
- Tobacco smoke exposure
- Cow- and soy-milk formula
- Processed food in maternal diet
- Low vitamin D

EXAMINATION

Physical examination is often normal. Expiratory wheezing (rhonchi) is the most frequent abnormality noted on examination, although it may be only heard on forced expiration or may be absent altogether. Wheezing is a finding that may also be heard in other pathologic conditions with similar complaints, including inducible laryngeal obstruction, respiratory infections, tracheomalacia, foreign body inhalation, and chronic obstructive pulmonary disease. Crackles and inspiratory wheezes are not typically features of asthma and may point to cardiac or upper airway pathologic condition, respectively. Clinicians may observe findings of allergic rhinitis or the presence of polyps on nasal examination.[5]

TESTING

In patients with respiratory symptoms characteristic of asthma, the diagnosis of asthma can be made by testing to confirm the limitation of expiratory airflow. Diagnostic testing is important to perform at initial presentation, as symptoms and airflow restriction may resolve spontaneously with or without treatment. For this reason, the diagnosis of asthma proves to be more difficult after treatment is initiated.[23]

Spirometry is preferred over peak expiratory flow (PEF) testing. Measurements of PEF testing may vary as much as 20% between devices, so it is important that the same device is used each time for testing if being used for diagnosis.[23]

Forced expiratory volume for 1 second (FEV1) remains the primary reading used for diagnosis of expiratory airway limitation. FEV1 may be reduced in many lung pathologic conditions and with poor technique or effort. Reduction of FEV1/forced vital capacity (FVC) also indicates limitation in expiratory airflow.[23]

Expiratory airflow limitation can be confirmed by the following[5]:

- Spirometry with positive bronchodilator reversibility: increase in FEV1 of greater than 12% predicted
- If spirometry is not available, PEF increase of 20% after bronchodilator challenge is consistent with asthma
- Variability of twice daily PEF testing over a 2-week period, average daily PEF variability greater than 13%
- Positive exercise challenge test, fall in FEV1 of greater than 12% predicted or PEF greater than 15%
- Excessive variation of lung function between visits, variation of FEV1 greater than 12% predicted or PEF greater than 15%

Objective testing is recommended to document airflow limitation for patients already taking controller treatment.

For patients with variable respiratory symptoms and confirmed variable airflow limitation, the diagnosis of asthma is confirmed.

For patients with variable respiratory symptoms present without documented airflow limitation while on treatment, repeat testing can be performed after withholding bronchodilator treatment according to the following guideline[5]:

- Short-acting beta-2 receptor agonist (SABA) greater than 4 hours
- Twice daily long-acting beta-2 receptor agonist (LABA)/inhaled corticosteroid (ICS) greater than 12 hours
- Once daily LABA/ICS greater than 24 hours

For patients with few or no symptoms and objective airflow limitation on spirometry, repeat testing after withholding bronchodilator therapy or stepping down controller treatment may be considered.[5]

- If symptoms emerge and spirometry demonstrates expiratory limitation, asthma is confirmed.
- If symptoms remain controlled or objective testing does not demonstrate limitation, consider discontinuing controller and monitor for 1 year.
- If symptoms are uncontrolled with persistent airflow limitation, escalate controller therapy for 3 months. If no response, deescalate controller therapy and consider referral.

ASSESSMENT OF DISEASE CONTROL

The hallmark of treatment of asthma relies on the assessment of disease control.[5,24–26] Objective data are used to classify disease and guide treatment and cover control of asthma-related symptoms and risk of complications. Symptom review should include wheezing, chest tightness, shortness of breath, and cough. Escalating asthma-related symptoms confer higher risk of acute exacerbation.

Symptom control:

- Daytime symptoms: frequency, triggers, response to daytime symptoms
- Nighttime symptoms: awakenings, poor sleep
- Rescue treatment use: frequency of rescue inhaler for symptom control
- Limitation on activity: missed school, limitation on physical activity

Morbidity risk:

- Exacerbations
  ○ ED/Urgent Care visits since last office visit
  ○ Hospitalizations
  ○ Viral illnesses
  ○ Asthma action plan in place
    ▪ Escalation in treatment
    ▪ Oral steroid need
- Lung function: FEV1, FEV1/FVC, PEF recordings compared with prior
- Treatment side effects: review height, growth velocity, dose and frequency of corticosteroid use (inhaled and oral)

Treatment:

- Inhaler technique: demonstration of use by patient
- Adherence: missed doses (AM vs PM), medication expiration
- Goals/concerns: patient and caregiver

Comorbidities:

- Allergic rhinitis: sneezing, nasal congestion, nasal obstruction, medications
- Atopic dermatitis: rash, pruritis affecting sleep, topical medication use
- Food allergy: confirmed food allergy risk factor for asthma-related mortality
- Obesity: Age-adjusted body mass index, diet, physical activity

ASSESSMENT OF DISEASE SEVERITY

Asthma severity is classified based on retrospective review of symptom control, treatment required to control symptoms and exacerbations, as well as degree of airflow limitation.[5,27,28] Mild asthma, moderate asthma, and severe asthma are differentiated by medication required for symptom control. Asthma is classified as intermittent if rescue treatment is used less than 2 times per week.

Mild asthma is controlled with as-needed SABA medication alone or in combination with low-dose ICS. In addition, asthma can be controlled with daily low-dose ICS or as-needed low-dose ICS-formoterol combination therapy, leukotriene receptor antagonist (LTRA), or chromone (cromolyn). Symptoms in mild asthma occur less than daily and are associated with minimal limitation in daily activity. FEV1 is greater than 80% predicted in mild asthma.

Moderate disease classification of asthma is asthma with symptom control with daily low-dose ICS-LABA treatment. Patients with moderate asthma experience symptoms on most days or are awaken with symptoms once a week or more.

Severe asthma encompasses disease requiring daily medium dose ICS-LABA or escalated therapy. Children with severe asthma exhibit symptoms on most days, are awaken with symptoms once a week, or have low lung function (FEV1 <60% predicted value). Daily activity is extremely limited in the severe asthmatic (**Table 1**).

Although patients with severe asthma and uncontrolled asthma may present clinically similar, it is important to differentiate between these, as treatment differs. Persistent symptoms and frequent exacerbations are more commonly related to uncontrolled disease and can be controlled with more simplicity. Studies have shown that improper use of inhaled medications is common and can be present in up to 80% of community patients. Suboptimal medication adherence may also present with persistent symptoms and frequent exacerbation of disease. In children with symptoms not improving with standard treatment strategies, further investigation is necessary. Alternative disease processes, including inducible laryngeal obstruction/vocal cord dysfunction, gastroesophageal reflux disease (GERD), cardiovascular disease, and poor cardiorespiratory fitness, should be explored. Uncontrolled comorbid conditions, such as GERD, rhinosinusitis, obesity, and obstructive sleep apnea, may present as severe disease. Ongoing exposure to irritants or sensitizing agents in the home or educational environment may also be present and represents reversible causes of respiratory symptoms.

Table 1
Summary of asthma severity

Disease Severity	Mild	Moderate	Severe
Controller	• SABA as needed • Low-dose ICS • ICS-formoterol as needed • LTRA • Chromone	• Daily low dose ICS-LABA	• Daily medium or high dose ICS-LABA • Escalation of treatment
Symptoms	Less than daily	Most days a week	Often daily
Night-time symptoms	None	1+ per week	Often daily
Activity limitation	None or minimal	Moderate	Severe
FEV1% predicted, %	>80	60–80	<60

TREATMENT

Medications used in the treatment of asthma can be classified in 3 domains: rescue medications, controller medications, and add-on medications, which are typically used only in severe asthma. Treatment algorithms for asthma are continuously evolving, and recent updates have led to changes in historical treatment paradigm. Treatment of asthma revolves around the reduction of asthma-related symptoms, reducing or eliminating the need for rescue medications, and reduction of disease-related morbidity.[5,27,28]

Beta-2 receptor agonists function at the adrenergic receptors of intracellular adenyl cyclase. This action results in the conversion of adenosine triphosphate to cyclic adenosine monophosphate (c-AMP). Increased c-AMP levels result in bronchial smooth muscle relaxation and inhibits hypersensitivity mediators from mast cells.[5]

Beta-2 agonists used in the treatment of asthma are divided into short-acting and long-acting beta agonists. These medications are supplied in a liquid or powder metered dose inhaler (MDI), liquid for use in a nebulizer, and oral liquid and tablets. Albuterol and its R-enantiomer, levalbuterol, are commercially available SABA in the United States, with onset of action within minutes and duration of 4 to 6 hours. There is insufficient evidence to suggest levalbuterol is more effective than albuterol. Albuterol remains the preferred reliever medication. The use of MDI with appropriate spacer device appears to be noninferior to nebulized albuterol. The use of a face mask in addition to spacer is recommended for children under the age of 4.[5,23]

Long-acting beta agonists are more lipophilic with longer duration of action, typically around 12 hours, and a variable onset of action. Extended-release albuterol tablet, formoterol inhalation, and salmeterol inhalation are available and approved for the treatment of asthma in the United States. These medications are often found in combination with an ICS. Because of its water solubility, formoterol has a similar (1–3 minute) onset to action as SABA medications, affording the ability to be used as an as-needed rescue medication as reflected by the 2020 Global Initiative for Asthma (GINA) management guidelines. Prior studies have demonstrated increased severe asthma exacerbations of LABA compared with placebo leading to a black box warning added to all drugs containing LABA. Newer studies have not demonstrated this risk and showed a significant decrease in exacerbation risk with LABA/ICS compared with ICS alone.[5,29]

Anticholinergic bronchodilators, such as ipratropium, are not recommended for routine use because of its longer onset of action and increased side-effect profile. There is, however, evolving evidence for its use for treatment of severe exacerbations in patients over the age of 5. Long-acting muscarinic antagonists (LAMA), such as tiotropium, may be used as add-on therapy in patients over the age of 11 in severe asthma or in cases of LABA intolerance.[25]

Methylxanthines, such as theophylline, are not recommended as first-line treatment of asthma.[5]

The hallmark of controller medications is ICS. Corticosteroids used in the treatment of asthma are analogues to endogenous glucocorticoid cortisol. The anti-inflammatory and immune suppression effects of these compounds through alteration of nuclear gene transcription are responsible for the mechanism of action for asthma control. This results in inhibition of proinflammatory mediators responsible in large part for the pathophysiology of asthma and includes macrophages, eosinophils, mast cells, lymphocytes, and dendritic cells. In addition, the inhibition of phospholipase A2 results in an inflammatory state. Glucocorticoids also inhibit expression of proinflammatory genes encoding for cyclooxygenase-2, inducible nitric oxide synthase, tumor necrosis factor-alpha, interleukins, prostaglandin, and leukotriene as well as reduction of neutrophil migration. Given the intracellular action, the effects of glucocorticoids persist longer than the presence in plasma.[5,29]

ICS are synthetic analogues of glucocorticoids, which are halogenated affording increased local potency without significantly increasing systemic effect. Because of the modifications of the parent molecule, changes in formulations confer variable effects and should be reviewed before prescription. In aerosolized formulations, spacer devices increase the amount of medication delivered to the lung tissue and decrease the amount deposited in the oropharynx or swallowed, as much as 40% to 90% of the actuated dose. Adverse effects include oropharyngeal candidiasis, dysphonia, coughing, and dose-related alteration of growth velocity, bone mineral density, and hypothalamus-pituitary-adrenal (HPA) axis function. Mouth rinsing with water may reduce some risks from oropharyngeal exposure. Overall, benefits of ICS therapy far outweigh risks.[29]

ICS therapy results in improved quality of life, improved lung function, reduced asthma symptoms, reduced frequency and severity of acute exacerbations, reduced asthma-related morbidity, reduced mortality, and a reduction in airway hyperreactivity and inflammation. ICS doses are differentiated in low, medium, and high doses, although comparison between different ICS medications and formulation is not straightforward. Most clinical benefit is seen at even low doses.[5,29]

Commercially available ICS medications in the United States include the following[5]:

- Beclomethasone
- Budesonide
- Ciclesonide
- Fluticasone
- Mometasone

Combined LABA-ICS medications have gained popularity in the treatment of asthma. As-needed low-dose ICS-formoterol combination therapy has more recently been shown to significantly reduce severe exacerbations among patients with mild asthma compared with SABA therapy and noninferior to routine ICS treatment. This effect is likely related to the increased hydrophilicity of formoterol with similar onset of action to commercially available SABA medications. In these instances, average ICS dose was lower in the ICS-formoterol group than routine ICS treatment groups. In more severe disease, GINA step 3 to 5, addition of LABA to ICS therapy resulted in improved clinical outcomes and reduction of severe exacerbations in patients aged 12 or older. ICS-formoterol therapy can be used as both controller and rescue treatment. Combining these 2 classes of medication in a combination inhaler increases compliance and has been seen to reduce hospitalization for severe exacerbation compared with separate LABA and ICS inhalers.[29-31]

Commercially available low-dose ICS-LABA for controller and rescue use include the following[5]:

- Beclomethasone-formoterol
- Budesonide-formoterol (USA)

Commercially available controller ICS-LABA for GINA step 3 to 5[5]

- Beclomethasone-formoterol
- Budesonide-formoterol (USA)
- Fluticasone-vilanterol (once daily) (USA)
- Fluticasone-formoterol

- Fluticasone-salmeterol (USA)
- Mometasone-formoterol (USA)

Systemic corticosteroids are used short term (<14 days) for acute severe exacerbation with the goal to prevent progression of exacerbation. Oral corticosteroids are preferred over parenteral doses because of given favorable side-effect profile, notably less mineralocorticoids effect and greater dose flexibility. Typical dosing is 1 to 2 mg/kg/d prednisolone (maximum of 40 mg) for 3 to 7 days. When treatment results in symptom and lung function improvement within 14 days of treatment, oral corticosteroid treatment may be discontinued abruptly. Long-term systemic corticosteroid therapy (duration longer than 14 days) may be required for more severe exacerbations or uncontrolled asthma. Adverse effects include osteoporosis, elevated blood pressure, HPA axis suppression, weight gain and obesity, skin thinning, cataracts, glaucoma, muscular weakness, insomnia, peptic ulcer, and avascular necrosis. Side effects of short-term therapy are typically reversible and uncommon.[5,32]

Leukotriene modifiers, such as montelukast, zafirlukast, and zileuton, are reserved for add-on use of patients taking daily ICS; however, they are less effective than the addition of LABA to therapy. Recently, the Food and Drug Administration has required a black box warning for montelukast encompassing neuropsychiatric events, including agitation, depression, sleep disturbance, and suicidality.[33]

Macrolide antimicrobials, such as azithromycin, are not generally recommended for pediatric asthma for chronic use or in acute exacerbation.[34]

Omalizumab, an anti-IgE monoclonal antibody, is an injectable add-on therapy approved for use in patients 6 years of age or older with severe allergic asthma not controlled with LABA-ICS therapy. Dosing is based on age and pretreatment serum IgE level. Treatment may result in improvement of quality of life, reduction of oral corticosteroid dose requirement, and reduced exacerbations.[35]

Anti–interleukin-5 medications (benralizumab, mepolizumab) target this cytokine, which is required for eosinophil function, and are approved for patients 12 years of age or older with severe eosinophilic asthma failing treatment with LABA-ICS therapy. These injectable therapies may reduce exacerbation frequency, reduce asthma-related symptoms, reduce oral steroid dose, and improve lung function.[36,37]

Dupilumab, anti-IL4 receptor alpha monoclonal antibody, is approved for treatment of severe eosinophilic asthma in patients aged 12 yeras or older who have failed treatment with LABA-ICS treatment. Therapy blocks interleukin-4 (IL-4) and IL-13 proinflammatory cytokines and similarly may result in reduction of exacerbations, oral corticosteroid dose, and improvement of quality of life, symptom control, and lung function.[38]

Figs. 1–3 outline the 2020 GINA stepwise treatment algorithm for patients 5 years of age and younger, 6 to 11 years of age, and 12 years and older, respectively.

MANAGEMENT OF ACUTE EXACERBATION

Acute exacerbations include acute and subacute worsening of lung function or asthma-related symptoms.[5] In the primary care setting, it is of utmost importance to triage the severity of exacerbation. Exacerbations can be graded as mild, moderate, severe, or life threatening.

Severe and Life-Threatening Exacerbations

- Symptoms may include the following:
  - Inability speak in full sentences
  - Use of accessory respiratory muscles

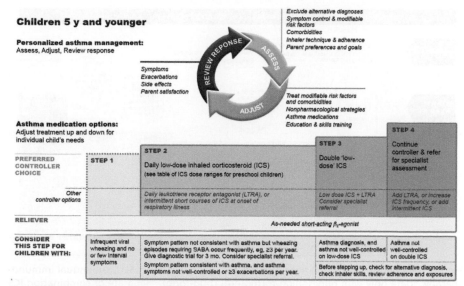

Fig. 1. Treatment of asthma under age 5. (GINA © 2020 Global initiative for Asthma, reprinted with permission. Available from www.ginasthma.org.)

- ○ Tachycardia
- ○ Tachypnea
- ○ Hypoxia with Spo₂ less than 94%
- ○ PEV less than 50% predicted
- • Treatment
  - ○ Short-acting beta-agonist (albuterol)
  - ○ Supplemental oxygen

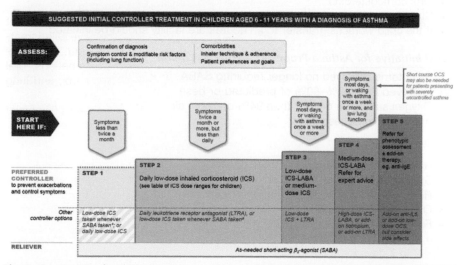

Fig. 2. Treatment of asthma age 6 to 11. OCS, oral corticosteroids. ᵃSeparate ICS and SABA inhalers. (GINA © 2020 Global initiative for Asthma, reprinted with permission. Available from www.ginasthma.org.)

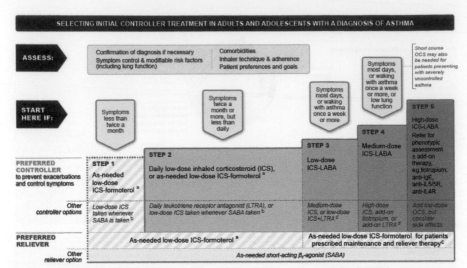

Fig. 3. Treatment of asthma in ages 12+. HDM, house dust mite; SLIT, sublingual immuno-therapy. [a]Data only with budesonide-formoterol (bud-form). [b]Separate or combination ICS and SABA inhalers. [c]Low-dose ICS-form is the reliever only for patients prescribed bud-form or BDP-form maintenance and reliever therapy. [d]Consider adding HDM SLIT for sensitized patients with allergic rhinitis and FEV1 >70% predicted. (GINA © 2020 Global initiative for Asthma, reprinted with permission. Available from www.ginasthma.org.)

- ○ Systemic corticosteroid medications
- ○ Transfer to acute care facility

Mild to Moderate Exacerbation

- SABA (nebulized or via inhaler and spacer 4–10 puffs every 20 minutes for 1 hour)
- Oral corticosteroids
- Supplemental oxygen to achieve a goal of 94% to 98% Spo_2
- If the child worsens, transfer to an acute care facility should be initiated

Global Initiative for Asthma-Proposed Discharge Criteria

- Symptoms improved no longer requiring SABA
- Improved PEF (60%–80% of predicted or best)
- Oxygen saturation greater than 94% on room air
- Adequate home resources

If these are met:

- Rescue SABA as needed
- Start or step up controller
- Review technique and adherence to treatment
- Oral steroid prescription
- Follow-up
  - ○ 1 to 2 days for children
  - ○ 2 to 7 days for adolescents

At follow-up:

- Are symptoms resolving?

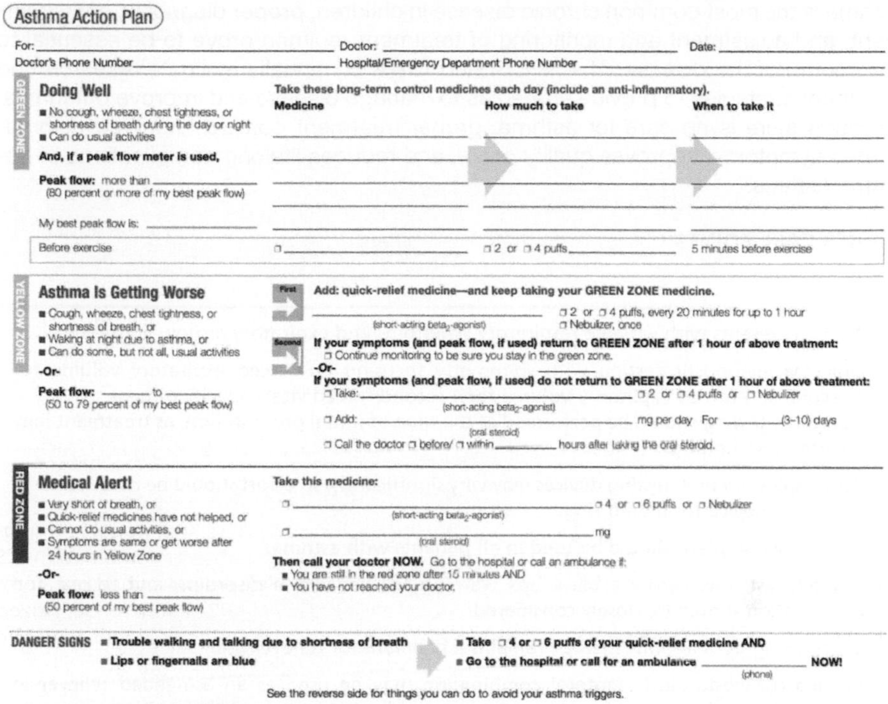
Asthma Action Plan

For: ______ Doctor: ______ Date: ______

Doctor's Phone Number ______ Hospital/Emergency Department Phone Number ______

GREEN ZONE

Doing Well

- No cough, wheeze, chest tightness, or shortness of breath during the day or night
- Can do usual activities

And, if a peak flow meter is used,

Peak flow: more than ______ (80 percent or more of my best peak flow)

My best peak flow is: ______

Take these long-term control medicines each day (include an anti-inflammatory).

Medicine	How much to take	When to take it
Before exercise ☐ ______	☐ 2 or ☐ 4 puffs ______	5 minutes before exercise

YELLOW ZONE

Asthma Is Getting Worse

- Cough, wheeze, chest tightness, or shortness of breath, or
- Waking at night due to asthma, or
- Can do some, but not all, usual activities

-Or-

Peak flow: ______ to ______ (50 to 79 percent of my best peak flow)

First: **Add: quick-relief medicine—and keep taking your GREEN ZONE medicine.**

______ (short-acting $beta_2$-agonist) ☐ 2 or ☐ 4 puffs, every 20 minutes for up to 1 hour ☐ Nebulizer, once

Second: **If your symptoms (and peak flow, if used) return to GREEN ZONE after 1 hour of above treatment:**

☐ Continue monitoring to be sure you stay in the green zone.

-Or-

If your symptoms (and peak flow, if used) do not return to GREEN ZONE after 1 hour of above treatment:

☐ Take: ______ (short-acting $beta_2$-agonist) ☐ 2 or ☐ 4 puffs or ☐ Nebulizer

☐ Add: ______ (oral steroid) mg per day For ______ (3–10) days

☐ Call the doctor ☐ before/ ☐ within ______ hours after taking the oral steroid.

RED ZONE

Medical Alert!

- Very short of breath, or
- Quick-relief medicines have not helped, or
- Cannot do usual activities, or
- Symptoms are same or get worse after 24 hours in Yellow Zone

-Or-

Peak flow: less than ______ (50 percent of my best peak flow)

Take this medicine:

☐ ______ (short-acting $beta_2$-agonist) ☐ 4 or ☐ 6 puffs or ☐ Nebulizer

☐ ______ (oral steroid) mg

Then call your doctor NOW. Go to the hospital or call an ambulance if:

- You are still in the red zone after 15 minutes AND
- You have not reached your doctor.

DANGER SIGNS

- **Trouble walking and talking due to shortness of breath**
- **Lips or fingernails are blue**

- **Take ☐ 4 or ☐ 6 puffs of your quick-relief medicine AND**
- **Go to the hospital or call for an ambulance** ______ (phone) **NOW!**

See the reverse side for things you can do to avoid your asthma triggers.

Fig. 4. Asthma action plan.

- Does oral steroid need to be continued?
- Continue SABA as needed
- Continue controller at higher dose for 1 to 2 weeks up to 3 months
- Assess for modifiable risk factors
- Asthma action plan in place, understood, or in need of adjustment
- Consider specialist referral for multiple yearly exacerbations

ASTHMA ACTION PLAN

Asthma action plans were introduced by the National Heart, Lung, and Blood Institute (NHLBI) (**Fig. 4**). The goal of an asthma action plan is to help patients and families manage intermittent symptoms that are seen with asthma. Asthma actions plans are a personalized strategy developed to facilitate early recognition and management of acute asthma exacerbations.[39]

Asthma action plans include the following:

- Daily medications
- Known triggers and strategies to control these factors
- Strategies to recognize escalating symptoms
- Treatment strategies for worsened symptoms
- Treatment strategies for when to seek additional care and contact information

SUMMARY

Asthma is an inflammatory chronic condition that involves the airways. Significant morbidity is associated with uncontrolled asthma, resulting in significant costs. As asthma is the most common chronic disease in children, proper diagnosis, early treatment, and adjustment and monitoring of treatment regimen prove to be essential to the control of the disease. The NHLBI and GINA continually evaluate research and treatment strategies to provide strategies to manage disease and improve outcomes. Although there is no cure for asthma, proper treatment confers improved asthma-related symptoms, improves quality of life, and reduces lifelong complications of pediatric asthma.

CLINICS CARE POINTS

- Asthma presents with variable respiratory symptoms and expiratory airflow limitation.
- Objective diagnostic testing with spirometry focusing on forced expiratory volume for 1 second and forced expiratory volume for 1 second/forced vital capacity or peak expiratory testing should be performed at the time of initial presentation, as treatment may reverse these findings.
- Peak expiratory flow testing devices may vary significantly, so effort should be made to use 1 peak flow device for monitoring.
- Asthma action plans should be used in all patients with asthma.
- Montelukast now carries a black box warning for behavioral disorders, and its use and continuation should be closely considered.
- Short-acting beta-agonist therapy remains a hallmark for reliever use.
- Inhaled corticosteroid-formoterol combination may be used as an as-needed reliever in therapeutic escalation and has been incorporated in newer treatment algorithms.

REFERENCES

1. Marketos SG, Ballas CN. Bronchial asthma in the medical literature of Greek antiquity. Available at: https://pubmed.ncbi.nlm.nih.gov/6757243/. Accessed October 30, 2020.
2. FastStats - Asthma. Centers for Disease Control and Prevention, Centers for Disease Control and Prevention 2020. Available at: www.cdc.gov/nchs/fastats/asthma.htm.
3. Asthma. Centers for Disease Control and Prevention. Centers for Disease Control and Prevention; 2020. Available at: www.cdc.gov/asthma/default.htm.
4. Holgate ST. A brief history of asthma and its mechanisms to modern concepts of disease pathogenesis. Allergy Asthma Immunol Res 2010;2(3):165–71.
5. Global Initiative for Asthma - Global Initiative for .... Available at: https://ginasthma.org/wp-content/uploads/2020/06/GINA-2020-report_20_06_04-1-wms.pdf. Accessed October 30, 2020.
6. Sinyor B. Pathophysiology of asthma. 2020. Available at: https://www.ncbi.nlm.nih.gov/books/NBK551579/. Accessed October 30, 2020.
7. Torgerson DG, Ampleford EJ, Chiu GY, et al. Meta-analysis of genome-wide association studies of asthma in ethnically diverse North American populations. Available at: https://pubmed.ncbi.nlm.nih.gov/21804549/.
8. Levin AM, Mathias RA, Huang L, et al. A meta-analysis of genome-wide association studies for serum total IgE in diverse study populations. J Allergy Clin Immunol 2013;131(4):1176–84.

9. Shrine N, Portelli MA, John C, et al. Moderate-to-severe asthma in individuals of European ancestry: a genome-wide association study. Lancet Respir Med 2019; 7(1):20–34.

10. Horwood LJ, Fergusson DM, Shannon FT. Social and familial factors in the development of early childhood asthma. Pediatrics 1985;75(5):859–68.

11. den Dekker HT, Sonnenschein-van der Voort AMM, de Jongste JC, et al. Early growth characteristics and the risk of reduced lung function and asthma: a meta-analysis of 25,000 children. J Allergy Clin Immunol 2016;137(4):1026–35.

12. Boulet LP. Asthma and obesity. Clin Exp Allergy 2013 Jan;43(1):8–21.

13. Wahn U, Lau S, Bergmann R, et al. Indoor allergen exposure is a risk factor for sensitization during the first three years of life. J Allergy Clin Immunol 1997; 99(6 Pt 1):763–9.

14. Hogaboam CM, Carpenter KJ, Schuh JM, et al. Aspergillus and asthma–any link? Med Mycol 2005;43(Suppl 1):S197–202.

15. Driscoll A, Arshad S, Bont L, et al. Does respiratory syncytial virus lower respiratory illness in early life cause recurrent wheeze of early childhood and asthma? Critical review of the evidence and guidance for future studies from a World Health Organization-sponsored meeting. 2020. Available at: https://www.ncbi. nlm.nih.gov/pmc/articles/PMC7049900/.

16. Di Cicco M, Sepich M, Ragazzo V, et al. Potential effects of E-cigarettes and vaping in pediatric asthma. Minerva Pediatrica 2020;72(5):372–82.

17. Lee SL, Wong WH, Lau YL. Association between air pollution and asthma admission among children in Hong Kong. Clin Exp Allergy 2006;36(9):1138–46.

18. Lee JY, Leem JH, Kim HC, et al. Effects of traffic-related air pollution on susceptibility to infantile bronchiolitis and childhood asthma: a cohort study in Korea. J Asthma 2018;55(3):223–30.

19. Brigham EP, Woo H, McCormack M, et al. Omega 3 and omega-6 intake modifies asthma severity and response to indoor air pollution in children. Available at: https://pubmed.ncbi.nlm.nih.gov/30922077/.

20. Litonjua A, Al E, von Mutius E, et al. Six-year follow-up of a trial of antenatal vitamin D for asthma reduction: NEJM. 2020. Available at: https://www.nejm. org/doi/full/10.1056/NEJMoa1906137.

21. O'Sullivan BP, James L, Majure JM, et al. Obesity-related asthma in children: a role for vitamin D. Pediatric Pulmonol 2020;56(2):354–61.

22. Wolsk HM, Harshfield BJ, Laranjo N, et al. Vitamin D supplementation in pregnancy, prenatal 25(OH)D levels, race, and subsequent asthma or recurrent wheeze in offspring: secondary analyses from the Vitamin D Antenatal Asthma Reduction Trial. J Allergy Clin Immunol 2017;140(5):1423–9.e5.

23. Graham BL. Standardization of spirometry 2019 update. An Official American Thoracic Society and European Respiratory Society Technical Statement. Available at: https://www.atsjournals.org/doi/10.1164/rccm.201908-1590ST.

24. Taylor DR, Bateman ED, Boulet LP, et al. A new perspective on concepts of asthma severity and control. Available at: https://pubmed.ncbi.nlm.nih.gov/ 18757695/.

25. Meltzer EO, Busse WW, Wenzel SE, et al. Use of the Asthma Control Questionnaire to predict future risk of asthma exacerbation. Available at: https:// pubmed.ncbi.nlm.nih.gov/21093024/.

26. Schatz M, Zeiger RS, Yang SJ, et al. The relationship of asthma impairment determined by psychometric tools to future asthma exacerbations. 2011. Available at: https://pubmed.ncbi.nlm.nih.gov/21868465/.

27. Reddel HK, Taylor DR, Bateman ED, et al. An official American Thoracic Society/ European Respiratory Society statement: asthma control and exacerbations: standardizing endpoints for clinical asthma trials and clinical practice. 2009. Available at: https://pubmed.ncbi.nlm.nih.gov/19535666/.
28. Chung K, Wenzel S, Brozek J, et al. International ERS/ATS guidelines on definition, evaluation and treatment of severe asthma. 2014. Available at: https://erj.ersjournals.com/content/43/2/343. Accessed December 28, 2020.
29. Williams DM. Clinical pharmacology of corticosteroids. Respiratory Care 2018; 63(6):655–70.
30. O'Byrne PM, FitzGerald JM, Bateman ED, et al. Inhaled combined budesonide-formoterol as needed in mild asthma. N Engl J Med 2018;378:1865–76.
31. Bateman ED, Reddel HK, O'Byrne PM, et al. As-needed budesonide-formoterol versus maintenance budesonide in mild asthma. N Engl J Med 2018;378: 1877–87.
32. Corticosteroids for preventing relapse following acute exacerbations of asthma. Available at: https://www.cochrane.org/CD000195/AIRWAYS_corticosteroids-for-preventing-relapse-following-acute-exacerbations-of-asthma.
33. Center for Drug Evaluation and Research. Boxed warning about mental health side effects for Singulair. Available at: https://www.fda.gov/drugs/drug-safety-and-availability/fda-requires-boxed-warning-about-serious-mental-health-side-effects-asthma-and-allergy-drug. Retrieved October 30, 2020.
34. Should macrolides be used for chronic asthma?. 2015. Available at: https://www.cochrane.org/CD002997/AIRWAYS_should-macrolides-be-used-chronic-asthma.
35. Henriksen DP, et al. Efficacy of omalizumab in children, adolescents, and adults with severe allergic asthma: a systematic review, meta-analysis, and call for new trials using current guidelines for assessment of severe asthma 2020. Available at: https://aacijournal.biomedcentral.com/articles/10.1186/s13223-020-00442-0.
36. Busse WW, Bleecker ER, FitzGerald JM, et al. Long-term safety and efficacy of benralizumab in patients with severe, uncontrolled asthma: 1-year results from the BORA phase 3 extension trial. 2019. Available at: https://pubmed.ncbi.nlm.nih.gov/30416083/.
37. Farne HA, Wilson A, Powell C, et al. Anti-IL5 therapies for asthma. 2017. Available at: https://pubmed.ncbi.nlm.nih.gov/28933516/.
38. Castro M, Al E, Harrington J, et al. Dupilumab efficacy and safety in moderate-to-severe uncontrolled asthma: NEJM. 2018. Available at: https://www.nejm.org/doi/full/10.1056/nejmoa1804092.
39. Asthma for Health Professionals. Available at: https://www.nhlbi.nih.gov/health-topics/asthma-for-health-professionals. Accessed November 02, 2020.

Gait Disorders

Margaret E. Gibson, MD[a],*, Natalie Stork, MD[b,c]

KEYWORDS

- Pediatric • Gait • Limp • Intoeing • Pes planus • Gait analysis • Movement
- Postural control

KEY POINTS

- Gait changes with age, so it is important to understand how normal gait develops in children.
- Changes in gait are a common reason for a parent to seek care for a child, but these are often normal variations warranting reassurance.
- Urgent conditions causing gait abnormalities or limping should be quickly identified and sent to the appropriate orthopedic provider for definitive diagnosis and treatment.
- Gait abnormalities may be the presenting finding of systemic conditions, so a broad differential diagnosis is important in evaluating and treating children with gait changes.

 Video content accompanies this article at http://www.primarycare.theclinics.com.

INTRODUCTION/HISTORY/DEFINITIONS/BACKGROUND

Changes in a child's gait pattern exist on a spectrum of normal variation to pathologic, some of which may require emergent medical attention. To know if a gait change is concerning one must first know how to assess gait and then be aware of normal variations in gait patterns. Gait tends to develop and mature just as other milestones that the primary care physician follows regularly in each patient. Understanding of this progression and how it can be affected by common childhood diseases is also important, as at times a gait change may be the presenting symptom of a more serious underlying condition.

[a] Department of Community and Family Medicine, University of Missouri Kansas City, Kansas City, MO, USA; [b] Department of Orthopaedics and Musculoskeletal Medicine, Childrens Mercy Hospital, 2401 Gillham Road, Kansas City, MO 64108, USA; [c] Orthopaedic Surgery, University of Missouri-Kansas City School of Kansas City, Kansas City, MO, USA
* Corresponding author. Truman Medical Center Lakewood, 7900 Lee's Summit Road, Kansas City, MO 64139.
E-mail address: margaret.gibson@tmcmed.org

Prim Care Clin Office Pract 48 (2021) 395–415
https://doi.org/10.1016/j.pop.2021.04.004
0095-4543/21/© 2021 Elsevier Inc. All rights reserved.

primarycare.theclinics.com

Normal Gait

A normal gait pattern should be smooth and fluid in nature and demonstrates predictable changes with age. A toddler gait pattern (12–16 months) has a wide base with short, fast strides. Children around 3 years of age show improved coordination; they have a more fluid gait with equal strides and reciprocal arm motion. Toddlers and young children usually have a flat foot to flat foot pattern of gait. By age 7 years all elements of a mature gait are present, including a heel to toe pattern, a longer stride, and decreased cadence.[1] Normal gait requires intact neurologic and musculoskeletal systems, including a normal motor cortex, proper alignment, a functioning skeleton, tendons, and muscles.[2]

The gait cycle can be characterized as a series of 4 actions that occur in a smooth orchestrated fashion—heel strike, toe off, swing, and heel strike.[3] This series of events is often divided into 2 phases: stance phase, which occurs when the foot is in contact with the ground, and swing phase, which occurs when the foot leaves the ground, progressing forward in space. During walking, 60% of the gait cycle is spent in stance and 40% in swing. The stance phase includes heel strike, midstance, and push off. During the swing phase at least one limb is non–weight-bearing. As speed increases, time in stance phase decreases.

Heel strike is when the back of the foot contacts the ground. Following heel strike, the subtalar joint pronates, allowing the foot to adapt and helping to absorb the impact. The subtalar joint then supinates during midstance and push-off, allowing the foot to function as a stable lever.[4]

OBSERVATION/ASSESSMENT/EVALUATION
History

The importance of history is emphasized during medical school, and this continues to be true when considering gait concerns. History will need to include information about gait changes or pain including location, onset, duration, trauma, modifying factors, and associated systemic signs or symptoms. Prior treatments, physician visits including any surgeries, and imaging related to the gait change should also be documented. Inquiring what the family's concerns and observations are regarding the gait pattern or chief complaint can provide particularly useful information. Ask if limb use and gait generally seem symmetric to the family. Ask if the child walks on tip toe or is flat footed. Find out how the child sits. Ask if it is in a W pattern.[5] Ask if other children or parents exhibited similar behaviors. Age is also extremely important to consider for both normal variation in gait patterns and pathologic gait patterns. Persistence of gait variation past various ages may be the first clue to a pathologic condition. In addition, certain diseases or pathology is more common in certain ages or stages of development.

Depending on the patient's age, the history may only be obtained from a parent or guardian, but whenever possible make sure to ask direct questions to the patient. Ask the parent or guardian about pregnancy, delivery, and the child's development. Assess whether the child has met the standard motor milestones. In general, children should sit without support around 6 to 7 months, they should be walking independently between 10 and 16 months, and running should present around 14 to 24 months.[6] Significant abnormalities in reaching these milestones may indicate abnormal development.

Family history should also be included during this part of the evaluation. Family history of autoimmune, rheumatologic, and neurologic diseases are especially important. Familial traits can alter gait and potentially reveal higher risk diseases.

Physical Examination

Pertinent vital signs include a temperature, height, and weight. It is important to compare the patient's height and weight to standard growth charts; if prior heights and weights are available for review a growth curve will help the assessment. Short stature or growth, −2 standard deviations for age and sex may indicate a systemic disorder or metabolic disease. Overweight or obese children are at an increased risk of tibia vara and slipped capital femoral epiphysis.

If possible, watch the patient walk to the examination room before the official visit with the physician begins. Watching the patient walk will be the best opportunity to see the true gait without the patient being aware he or she is being examined. As you walk into the room assess the child; does he or she seem to be ill or in severe pain? How does the child move in the examination room, for example, how does he/she climb on the stool, chair, or examination table, is he/she using limbs similarly?

A good musculoskeletal examination follows the same formula with each complaint: inspection; palpation; range of motion; strength; special testing; and a neurovascular examination. When considering gait abnormalities, the bench physical examination helps to characterize the gait pattern. Inspection and range of motion are a good starting point for the initial examination, with other parts of the examination varying depending on the involved areas.[7]

Inspection

Inspection evaluates for swelling, bruising, rashes, wounds, muscle wasting, or deformities and then assesses for angulation and rotation. When assessing gait, it is important to be able to see the lower extremities. A thorough examination is conducted with the patient barefoot and the lower extremities visible to the midthigh. Begin with standing alignment and walking. Have the patient stand with the knees straight ahead and arms at the sides.

Stand in front of the patient and assess frontal alignment with the patella facing forward looking a "knock-kneed" or "bow-legged" appearance. Genu valgum (knock-knee) can be assessed by looking at the intermalleolar distance, and genu varum (bow-leg) can be assessed by examining the intercondylar distance at the knee. These measurements can be conducted lying down, especially in younger children who may be more comfortable on a parent's lap (**Fig. 1**).

Gait differences related to rotational variation or deformity is assessed by observing the child walking and with your bench examination. Tripping, falling, and cosmetic

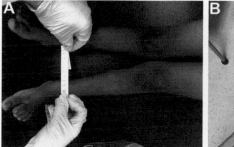
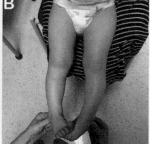

Fig. 1. (*A*) Genu valgum (knock-knee, observe/measure intermalleolar distance). (*B*) Genu varum (bow-leg, observe/measure intercondylar distance). ([*A*] *Courtesy of* James Weihe, MD, Kansas City, MO.)

abnormalities are often concerns of parents in children younger than 4 years with rotational findings.[8]

Hip rotation can be assessed with the child prone and the knees flexed to right angles. Rotate the legs to determine the internal and external rotation (**Fig. 2**). Hip rotation should be symmetric, and on average, there is approximately 50° of internal rotation and 45° of external rotation. Internal rotation in girls is usually 10° greater. Femoral anteversion is determined by increased internal rotation of the femoral neck in relation to the femoral condyles. Clinically, this manifests as increased internal rotation of the hips relative to external rotation. With regard to internal rotation, 70° is mild, 80° is moderate, and 90° is severe.[9] In contrast, when internal rotation is limited, especially if unilateral or asymmetrically limited, that can be an indication of intraarticular hip pathology, such as slipped capital femoral epiphysis, or hip effusion.

Rotation of the tibia or lower portion of the leg, tibial torsion is assessed by looking at the thigh-foot angle. This angle describes the rotation of the tibia and the hindfoot in relation to the longitudinal axis of the thigh. The child will need to be prone, flex the knees to 90°, and examine the foot (**Fig. 3**). With internal tibial torsion there will be a negative thigh-foot angle, which often manifests as intoeing. In contrast with external tibial torsion, the thigh-foot angle will be positive and may correspond with an out-toed gait pattern. The average thigh-foot angle is around 10° in most patients.[10] The tibia externally rotates during growth; therefore, internal tibia torsion tends to improve over time.

The foot progression angle or gait angle is a key component in assessing for rotational variation or deformity. This is assessed when the child walks in a straight line toward you or the observer and is the angle made by the foot to the floor, in the line of progression toward you (**Fig. 4**). Intoeing is documented as a negative angle and out-toeing a positive angle. Slight intoeing to −5° is normal.[11] Classify the foot type as neutral, pronated, or supinated. If the forefoot seems adducted, then flexibility will need to be assessed.

The arch of the foot should be assessed with the child non–weight-bearing and weight-bearing. The foot may seem to have a normal arch when seated, but when

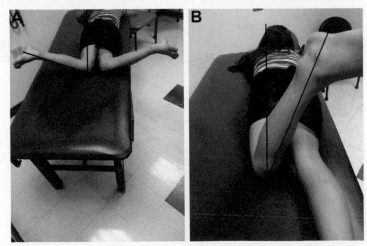

Fig. 2. (*A*) Hip internal rotation (IR)—IRangle, femoral anteversion (∼70°). (*B*) External rotation (ER)—ER angle, femoral anteversion; the difference between IR and ER is 30° or greater (ER ∼30°).

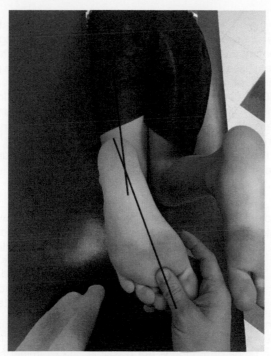

Fig. 3. Thigh-foot angle, measurement for internal tibial torsion.

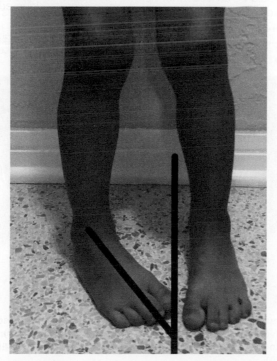

Fig. 4. Foot progression angle.

the patient stands the arch may completely flatten out. If you look at the heels of the patient with flat feet you will notice the hindfoot or calcaneus is in valgus relative to the leg. If a patient demonstrates pes planus (flat footed), have them stand on their toes (**Fig. 5**A). As a patient rises on their toes, with flexible flat foot (flexible pes planovalgus) you will see the hindfoot or heel transition into varus, and the patient will develop a visible arch (**Fig. 5**B). A flat foot that does not develop an arch, and in which the hindfoot or heel remains in valgus or does not move when the patient stands on their toes, is a rigid flat foot and is pathologic. A stiff flat foot can be painful and may be due to underlying abnormality, such as tarsal coalition. It is important for the physician or clinician to recognize that flat feet are common in infancy and young children, with the natural arch developing throughout the first decade of life.[12]

Palpation

Palpation is to guide the examiner to the location of pain. A joint above and below the area of pain or deformity should be considered. At times with gait changes the child may not complain of pain in one joint and in those situations examine the back, hip, knee, ankle, and foot. Palpation should include the bones and associated soft tissues.[7]

Range of Motion

Range of motion includes the motion at each joint and rotational evaluation. Range of motion can be assessed in the active (patient driven) and passive (examiner driven) states. If full active range of motion is not possible, the examiner should determine if passively they can obtain a greater range. If muscle tone is high or spasticity is present, this can limit range of motion and may indicate a neurologic condition.

The hip joint should be assessed for flexion, extension, adduction, abduction, and internal and external rotation. Normal knee range of motion ranges from −5 to 15° of hyperextension to 130 to 140° of flexion.[13] Ankle joint movement is best assessed with the child prone, knees flexed to 90° (**Fig. 6**). In this position ankle dorsiflexion is

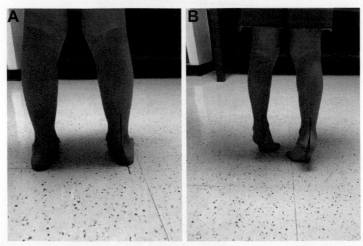

Fig. 5. (*A*) Pes planus (flat foot). Hindfoot valgus with the calcaneus (hindfoot) falling into valgus angle relative to the ankle. (*B*) Flexible pes planovalgus; as the patient arises on tip toes, an arch develops and the hindfoot (calcaneus) moves into varus relative to prior valgus positioning (Fig. 5A).

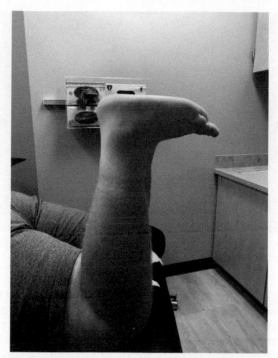

Fig. 6. Ankle range of motion, assessed with patient prone, knees flexed to 90°. This patient presented with decreased dorsiflexion on the affected side after an acute ankle injury.

not influenced by the gastrocnemius and hamstrings. The ankle should also be assessed for inversion, eversion, supination, and pronation.[14]

Strength

Strength assessment includes evaluation of the major muscle groups in the lower extremity. Assess tone and then perform manual muscle testing and grade on a 0 to 5 scale.[15] Neurovascular assessment requires solid understanding of the blood supply and innervation of the lower extremity. Lower extremity deep tendon reflexes, and Babinski reflexes should be assessed.

Special Testing

Special testing will be dictated by the location or pain or an injury to a certain location. There are some common tests that the examiner should be comfortable performing and interpreting. Check for Trendelenburg sign. Stand behind the patient. Ask the patient to stand on one leg and lift the other leg up off the floor. A positive test indicating weak hip abductors will show the pelvis dropping toward the elevated leg. Leg length discrepancy is determined by measuring the length from the hip to the knee and the knee to the ankle in the supine position. Galeazzi sign also assesses leg length. The patient lies on their back with their hips and knees bent; if the knees are not the same height a leg length discrepancy is likely present.

Imaging

Radiographs can be obtained to evaluate bony pathology. For leg length discrepancy, full limb radiographs OR a scanogram is recommended (**Fig. 7**). Further cross-

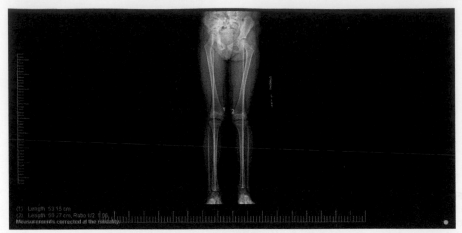

Fig. 7. Standing bilateral lower extremity radiographs for leg length discrepancy show a 2.88 cm difference.

sectional imaging computed tomography (CT) or MRI is often most helpful when the ordering physician or licensed medical professional has a specific diagnosis in mind (coalition, avascular necrosis, bone stress injury) or in the context of surgical planning. CT can help identify osseous abnormalities that are not seen on radiographs. MRI will better evaluate soft tissues. If infection, tumor, or synovitis is a concern, this type of advanced imaging with and without contrast can be helpful.[16,17]

DISCUSSION
Common Variations in Toddlers and Children

Once children start walking some variations are commonly seen by the primary care provider, and it is important to understand which are normal and which may need referral for orthopedic evaluation. Unnecessary referrals cause stress for parents and can delay appointments for patients with more urgent conditions. It has been reported that up to half of new referrals to pediatric orthopedic clinics are for children with normal variations in the lower extremities.[18] Primary care providers who have a good understanding of common variants limit unnecessary tests and referrals and can provide reassurance to these patients and families.

Parents may be concerned that their child looks bowlegged as they start to walk. Physiologic bowing (genu varum) will seem symmetric and involve the femur and tibia. It usually resolves by 2 years of age. It is extremely common and benign. The child will have a history of normal development, the family history will usually be negative, and a screening examination should be normal, with the patient standing or lying down and the feet together, and the intercondylar distance should be less than or equal to 6 cm.[19] If the deformity has not resolved by 2 years of age, the varus deformity is asymmetric or increasing, or the height is less than the 25th percentile, obtain an anteroposterior (AP) radiograph of bilateral lower extremities, which includes the pelvis and the ankle mortise bilaterally[20] (**Fig. 8A**). This radiograph will help determine severity and if rickets or bony dysplasia need to be considered. Bowing also needs to be differentiated from tibia vara.

Tibia vara, or Infantile Blount disease, results from abnormal growth of the proximal medial tibial physis, usually develops in infancy, and presents around 2 years of age

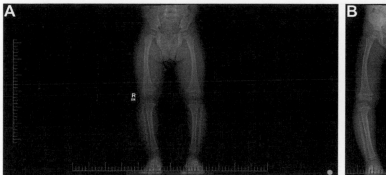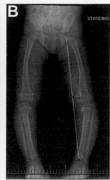

Fig. 8. (*A*) Physiologic genu varum on radiographs. (*B*) Tibia vara on radiographs: note the changes at the proximal tibial physis compared with Fig. 8A. The right proximal tibia demonstrates milder "beaking" with some sclerosis, whereas the left demonstrates significant deformity of the proximal tibia. The line drawn from the center of the left femoral head to the center of the distal tibial epiphysis represents the mechanical axis. This is where the weight is distributed with weight-bearing. This line should fall through the middle of the joint. ([*A*] *Courtesy of* James Welhe, MD, Kansas City, MO.)

(**Fig. 8**B). Risk factors include obesity and African American ethnicity. In addition, patients commonly have a history of early walking, when younger than 10 months. Clinically, infantile Blount disease often presents as pronounced genu varum persisting after 2 years of age. The gait pattern may reveal a lateral thrust of the knee through stance phase. Diagnosis is made by radiographs with characteristic features of "beaking" of the proximal medial tibia. Blount disease is characterized using the Lagenskiold classification to describe severity of the deformity based on radiographic appearance.[21] The natural history of the disease is poor, with progression leading to joint deformity, limb shortening, gait disturbance, and osteoarthritis. Pediatric orthopedic evaluation is recommended for these patients.

Intoeing and out-toeing are common concerns that parents bring to the children's primary care doctor (**Table 1**). Most of these will improve or resolve spontaneously, and observation is appropriate. Even if mild intoeing persists it rarely results in functional deficits or changes in activities of daily living or athletics. Intoeing can often be explained by one of more of the following orthopedic causes: metatarsus adductus, internal tibial torsion, and/or increased femoral anteversion.

Metatarsus adductus (MTA) is medial deviation of the forefoot in relation to the hind foot. It may be caused by intrauterine position, although true cause is unknown. MTA often resolves by 12 months of age. In children with a flexible deformity (forefoot easily corrects with gentle abduction of the forefoot), and normal ankle and subtalar range of motion, observation is appropriate. Stretching exercises are often discussed with the family, although evidence of the efficacy of home stretching exercises is sparse. Orthopedic referral is warranted for patients with a stiff or rigid deformity or one persisting beyond 4 to 6 months of age, as casting may be beneficial.[22]

The most common cause of intoeing in young children is internal tibial torsion. It is more common on the left side and seen equally in boys and girls. Children usually present between 2 and 4 years of age. Parents may note the child is clumsy or trips and falls frequently. When walking the clinician will note the patella faces forward, but the toes rotate inward. Similarly, on examination, when the patella is positioned pointing straight ahead, the toes rotate inward (**Fig. 9**). Another common examination finding

Table 1
Intoeing and out-toeing

	Intoeing	Special Consideration	Out Toeing	Special Consideration
Foot	Metatarsus adductus	Commonly diagnosed in infancy Affects forefoot Normal ankle ROM	Positional calcaneovalgus	Excessive dorsiflexion Foot may be positioned next to the shin Will correct spontaneously within a few months
	Clubfoot	Commonly diagnosed shortly after birth Rigid deformity of foot/ankle Rare deformity	Congenital vertical talus	Rigid deformity of foot Rocker-bottom deformity Does not improve on its own
	Skewfoot	Foot has serpentine appearance Normal ankle ROM	Pes planus	Almost universally present in children before school age Commonly bilateral May have associated Achilles tendon contracture
Tibia	Internal tibial torsion	Most common cause of intoeing between ages 15 mo and 4 y	External tibial torsion	Can present at any age May progress some with growth/age
Femur	Excessive femoral anteversion	Commonly presents between 4 and 7 y Female > Male Internal rotation of hips in EXCESS of external rotation by 45° or more	External rotation contracture of hips Femoral retroversion Slipped capital femoral epiphysis	Often presents in toddlers Improves spontaneously Bilateral Commonly presents in overweight/obese children Painless Overweight/obese Male Pain (hip/thigh/knee)

Abbreviation: ROM, range of motion.

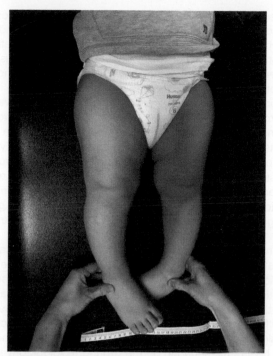

Fig. 9. Internal tibial torsion, the most common cause of intoeing.

is a negative thigh-foot angle with the child prone. Spontaneous improvement usually occurs over until around age 5 years; however, patients can continue to demonstrate residual internal tibial torsion beyond this age. In an otherwise typically developing child, internal tibial torsion generally does not affect function. Referral is considered for persistent deformity in children older than 8 years WITH significant functional impairment, those with a functional disability, or those with a thigh-foot angle greater than 15°.[23]

Femoral anteversion or antetorsion is common in girls, symmetric, and presents often with inward/medially rotated patella and feet. Parents will often note the patient sits in a "W" and has an abnormal running pattern.[5] Intoeing is seen in patients with femoral anteversion most noticeable between ages 4 and 7 years. The femur is rotated on its long axis, and on examination there is increased hip internal rotation and decreased external rotation. Assess femoral rotation with the child on his/her stomach and knees flexed to 90°. Femoral anteversion is significant if the internal rotation is greater than 70°, and there is reduced external rotation[10] (see **Fig. 3**, Video 1). For mild cases observation and reassurance is appropriate.

Out-toeing can be seen with femoral retroversion, external tibial torsion, and flat feet (see later discussion). However, an acute change with an increased and asymmetric out-toed gait pattern can be seen with slipped femoral capital epiphysis, acute injury to the affected lower extremity, as well as after patients have been immobilized in a walking boot or cast for a period of time.

External tibial torsion may progress with growth, as the tibia rotates laterally. It often presents in children 4 to 7 years old. External tibial torsion may be associated with knee pain, thought to occur due to malalignment of the patellofemoral joint. This external tibial torsion has been seen more commonly in combination with excessive femoral anteversion or antetorsion. Correction of rotational variation often involves an osteotomy, which is not without risk. Literature regarding definitive long-term sequela or functional disability of more extreme rotational variations is sparse. Surgical intervention is often reserved for those individuals with significant functional limitations and or pain refractory to nonoperative measures.

Genu valgum, or knock-knee alignment, commonly presents between 2 and 4 years of age, peaking around 3 to 4 years of age (see **Fig. 1**A). In addition to general inspection and grossly noting genu valgum, you can objectively measure genu valgum by measuring the intermalleolar distance with the child standing or lying down, up to 8 cm is generally physiologic in nature.[20,24] Management initially involves observation and parental reassurance. If the deformity persists over 8 year of age, is severe, or there is associated pain, then referral to a pediatric orthopedist may be warranted for possible surgical intervention.[19] It is commonly seen in obese girls in late childhood.[25] It can aggravate patellofemoral instability or contribute to knee pain pending severity.

Leg length discrepancy (LLD) can manifest as a change in gait. It can be anatomic or due to a functional deformity. A skeletal maturity of difference of greater than 2 cm is considered significant, but gait deviations have been noted with discrepancies starting at 1 cm.[26] Patients may present with back or leg pain, stress fractures, or osteoarthritis. Pending the severity of LLD, different gait patterns can be seen. Patients may demonstrate a shift in weight (subtle fall) toward the short leg while circumducting the longer leg. With significant LLD, patients may walk on the toes of the shorter leg, unable to place the heel of the short leg on the ground. Radiography is considered the gold standard and includes full limb radiographs, scanograms, and computerized digital radiographs.[27]

Foot

A flat foot is one with a loss of the medial longitudinal arch. Children often present with "flat feet" before 4 years of age because the arch is obscured by the plantar fat pad and the foot seems flat. Flat feet are usually due to ligamentous laxity. Improvement is often seen after the first year of walking. Children who present with painless flat feet do not require intervention. When weight-bearing there is no arch visible, but when the patient stands on tiptoe the arch is visible (see **Fig. 5**).

Excessive pronation of the foot does cause it to stay in a flexible position and not function as a firm lever. The foot flattens with weight-bearing and requires the muscles of the leg to raise the arch and stabilize the subtalar joint. It can overload the medial tibia and can lead to increased internal rotation of the tibia and patellar tracking abnormalities.

A rigid flat foot is pathologic and may be the result of a tarsal coalition, navicular osteochondrosis, infection, arthritis, or tumor. Subtalar motion may be limited, and an arch will not appear when the child stands on tiptoe. Radiographs or advanced imaging can help in the diagnosis of these conditions.

Excessive supination is seen with high-arched cavus feet and tends to be more rigid. It is stable for push-off but does not absorb shock well and may result in stress injuries most commonly of the fifth metatarsal. A high-arched foot may be on the spectrum of normal variation but may be a clue to an underlying neurologic disorder, such as Charcot-Marie-Tooth syndrome.

Toe walking, walking with a lack of heel strike, is due to plantar flexion at the ankle. It can be idiopathic or caused by tight or short heel cords, limb length discrepancies, club foot, and neurologic causes, such as cerebral palsy. It is a common variation of normal gait development, but if it persistent after 2 to 3 years of age referral to orthopedics is recommended.[28]

Limp

Parents may bring a child in for evaluation due to an inability to bear weight or a new limp. A limp is a deviation from the normal gait pattern. It will not be smooth, rather the gait will be uneven or jerky. Limp can present with associated pain or in some cases be pain free. Some causes are benign, but there are some cases that will need urgent orthopedic evaluation. A thorough history and physical examination is important in these cases and laboratory testing and imaging may help in making these diagnoses. Initial laboratory tests should look for infection and include a complete blood count (CBC), erythrocyte sedimentation rate (ESR), C-reactive protein (CRP), and blood cultures. These tests can help evaluate for infection, inflammatory arthritis, or neoplasm. Initial imaging should include radiographs. If there is limited range of motion, usually hip abduction and internal rotation, this raises concern for intraarticular pathology including potential hip effusion. Ultrasonography has an extremely high sensitivity in evaluating for the presence of a hip effusion. MRI best visualizes soft tissue, cartilage, joints, and bone edema. CT has little value in the initial evaluation but does reveal fine bone abnormalities.[29]

Types of Limp

If there is pain in one leg the patient may shorten the stance phase on that leg and present with an antalgic gait. An antalgic gait is commonly seen in the setting of acute trauma or bone stress injury, infection, or sometimes in the early stages of avascular necrosis (Table 2).

A nonantalgic or nonpainful gait pattern carries a wide differential, including hip subluxation or dislocation in the setting of hip dysplasia, later stages of Legg-Calve-Perthes, bone dysplasia, or neurologic cause. A steppage gait pattern is seen in neurologic conditions when the foot cannot dorsiflex, either due to weakness or due to limited range of motion, such as Charcot-Marie-Tooth and cerebral palsy (CP). The hip and knee must flex excessively for the foot to clear the ground during the swing phase. Circumduction gait is seen with neurologic conditions causing a stiff knee or ankle, such as in CP, as well as in patients with leg length discrepancy. The knee can be extended or hyperextended, and the leg must swing out and around so the foot clears the ground. An equinus gait pattern is when the child walks on their toes. Causes of equinus are multiple and include cerebral palsy, club foot, leg length discrepancy, tight Achilles, fractures, or injury to lower extremity or foot, including foreign body. A Trendelenburg gait is characterized by weakness of the hip abductors. The patient will demonstrate a shift or fall in the pelvis to the unaffected side during the swing phase (Video 2). It can be seen in developmental hip dysplasia, Legg-Calve-Perthes, slipped capital femoral epiphysis, muscular dystrophy, and hemiplegic cerebral palsy.[30]

Urgent or emergent causes of limp include hip joint infection (septic arthritis), osteomyelitis, diskitis (reviewed under infections), slipped capital femoral epiphysis (SCFE), compartment syndrome, which may have an associated open fracture or vascular compromise, toddler's fracture, and leukemia (reviewed under malignancy).

SCFE is the most common hip disorder in adolescents and requires emergent orthopedic treatment. The femoral head displaces in relation to the femoral neck (ice cream falls off the cone); this is seen in children often aged between 10 and 15 years with an increased body mass index. The highest prevalence is in African American boys. A patient may present with a limp and/or leg pain (at the knee or hip). On

Table 2
Limp

Gait	Pattern	Causes
Antalgic	Shortened stance phase due to pain on affected side	Urgent: infection, slipped capital femoral epiphysis (SCFE), compartment syndrome, acute trauma such as fracture Other: transient synovitis of the hip, developmental dysplasia of the hip, Legg-Calve-Perthes disease, systematic diseases such as rheumatoid or neuromuscular causes, trauma causing acute knee pathology including internal joint damage (meniscus tears, osteochondral defects), limb-length discrepancy, tarsal coalition, and overuse injuries
Nonantalgic		
Steppage	Lack foot dorsiflexion, hip and knee must flex excessively	Charcot-Marie-Tooth and CP
Circumduction	Knee is hyperextended and the leg must swing out	Leg-length discrepancy and CP
Equinus	Toe walking gait	CP, club foot, leg length discrepancy, tight Achilles, fractures, or injury including foreign body
Trendelenburg	Pelvis falls to the unaffected side during the swing phase due to weak hip abductors on the affected side	Developmental hip dysplasia, Legg-Calve-Perthes, slipped capital femoral epiphysis, muscular dystrophy, and hemiplegic cerebral palsy

Abbreviation: CP, cerebral palsy.

examination there is often a lack of internal rotation and abduction of the hip due to pain. Radiographs of the hip should be done immediately (AP *AND* frog leg) (**Fig. 10**). Once a diagnosis is made the patient should be made non–weight-bearing and sent to the emergency department. It is common to also have abnormality of the contralateral hip so bilateral imaging and surgery may be warranted.[31]

Compartment syndrome is a true orthopedic emergency. An influx of fluid into a fascial compartment leads to increased tissue pressure, resulting in decreased perfusion pressure and muscle and nerve ischemia. Fractures and soft tissue injuries are the most common causes of compartment syndrome. In children acute compartment syndrome is usually seen in the lower extremities and can therefore alter gait. The classic teaching of the 5 Ps (pain, paresthesia, paralysis, pallor, and pulselessness) associated with compartment syndrome may not present clearly in children, and it may be better to assess the 3 As (increasing analgesic requirement, anxiety, and agitation).[32] Diagnosis can be confirmed by compartment pressure testing, and treatment is emergent fasciotomy.

Toddler's fracture, a nondisplaced, spiral, or oblique fracture of the distal tibia, presents in children 9 months to 3 years of age.[33] The child will usually present with a limp or inability to bear weight. A rotational mechanism is most common; often there will only be a history of minor trauma, potentially and unwitnessed fall with a sibling or toy. Physical examination findings can include warmth to touch and pain with passive dorsiflexion of the ankle. Initial radiographs may be normal but repeat imaging in 1 to 2 weeks may show periosteal reaction and healing (**Fig. 11**).

Less urgent causes of limp include transient synovitis of the hip, developmental dysplasia of the hip, Legg-Calve-Perthes disease, systematic diseases such as rheumatoid or neuromuscular causes (see later discussion), knee pathology including internal joint damage (meniscus tears, osteochondral defects), limb-length discrepancy, tarsal coalition, and overuse injuries (Osgood-Schlatter, severs, and stress fractures).

Transient synovitis of the hip is a diagnosis of exclusion but a common one in children. These children aged 3 to 8 years are usually afebrile, will not seem terribly ill, and will have less severe pain with joint movement than those with septic arthritis. Often there was a viral illness within the last month. If a child can bear weight and has a CRP less than 20 mg/L the chance of septic arthritis is 1%.[34]

Developmental dysplasia of the hip is usually identified in newborns with hip instability. Strong risk factors include female gender, family history, and breech presentation. Other risk factors include those that may affect the intrauterine environment, such as first born, oligohydramnios, or twin gestation. Acetabular dysplasia and hip subluxation can present in children who are walking with as limp, joint pain, and osteoarthritis. When presenting in children of walking age surgical intervention is usually required and referral to an orthopedic surgeon is recommended.[35]

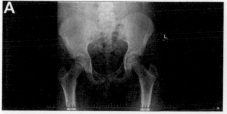 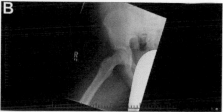

Fig. 10. A 12-year-old boy presented with a limp for 3 weeks and was found to have a slipped capital femoral epiphysis on the right hip. Findings are subtle on these radiographs. (*A*) AP view of the pelvis and (*B*) lateral view of the frog leg

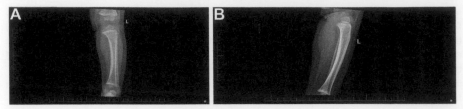

Fig. 11. AP (*A*) and lateral (*B*) radiographs of the tibia and fibula demonstrate a Toddler's fracture of the tibia.

Legg-Calve-Perthes disease is idiopathic avascular necrosis of capital femoral epiphysis. Patients who present with Legg-Calve-Perthes disease tend to be younger than those who present with SCFE. The presenting gait may be a lurch gait (during the stance phase the body leans to the affected side) or a stiff hip gait (the pelvis and lower back swing the whole leg, rather than the hip flexors bringing the leg through).[36] Physical examination will reveal pain with internal rotation and flexion. Radiographs will show mild flattening of the femoral head, sclerosis, and a crescent sign (**Fig. 12**). Often an AP of the pelvis is helpful to have a comparison view of the opposite femoral head. Referral to an orthopedic specialist is recommended for ongoing management. Children younger than 6 years of can usually be managed nonoperatively. In older children surgical intervention may be required.[37]

Limps associated with acute knee pathology may have a history of recent trauma. Examination may reveal an effusion or limited range of motion, and special testing such as the anterior and posterior drawer, Lachman, McMurray, and Thessaly tests should be performed. Radiographs can help evaluate for fracture and osteochondral defects. Osteochondral defects are often best seen on a tunnel or notch view. MRI can help confirm intraarticular pathology in the setting of an effusion. Referral for definitive treatment is recommended for osteochondral defect, fracture, or ligamentous instability. A limp and associated effusion in the absence of trauma or injury should raise suspicion for rheumatologic or infectious cause.[38]

Abnormal Gait Caused by Special Conditions

Infection

The most concerning pediatric musculoskeletal infections are osteomyelitis and septic arthritis. If the infection is in the lower extremity this can lead to a gait change or pain with walking. Although acute presentation does occur often, the onset may be insidious, requiring the clinician to be vigilant. If hardware is present from prior orthopedic surgical procedures the risk of infection is higher.

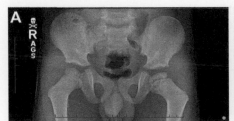
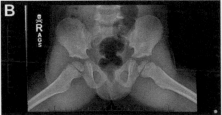

Fig. 12. AP (*A*) and bilateral frog leg (*B*) radiographs demonstrate Legg-Calve-Perthes of the left hip. (*Courtesy of* James Weihe, MD, Kansas City, MO.)

Osteomyelitis is a seeding of bacteria into the bone and usually occurs through hematogenous spread in children. The child will usually present with fever, warmth, edema, diffuse bone pain, and refusal to bear weight or change in limb usage. Plain radiographs may show deep soft tissue swelling. MRI is the preferred imaging modality. Laboratory evaluation should include a CBC, ESR, CRP, and blood cultures. Treatment involves appropriate antibiotics, and surgery is not always required.

Septic arthritis is an intraarticular joint infection, which is a surgical emergency. Presentation includes pain, limp, and possible fever. Examination will illicit pain with active and passive joint range of motion. Obtain a CBC, ESR, and CRP. Then the Kocher criteria can help with diagnosis, which includes an inability to bear weight, fever greater than 101.3°F, white blood count (WBC) greater than 12,000 per mm^3, and ESR greater than 40 mm/h. Joint fluid aspiration can be done for Gram staining, culture, and cell count (**Table 3**). Treatment is usually early initiation of antistaphylococcal antibiotics and surgical incision and drainage[16] (**Fig. 13**).

Diskitis and vertebral osteomyelitis can lead to limp or refusal to walk and will have associated back pain. A psoas abscess can present with gait changes, and the patient will have abdominal pain. A positive psoas sign is when the child lies on his or her back and the examiner passively extends the hip causing pain.

Neuromuscular
Cerebral palsy (CP) is the most prevalent neuromuscular disorder in children and the most common cause of chronic childhood disability.[39] There is usually a history of premature birth or perinatal distress. It is a nonprogressive upper motor neuron disease. In patients with CP the damage to the motor cortex can cause many changes to the muscles, including loss of control, abnormal tone, imbalance between agonists and antagonists, and primitive reflex patterns. Gait cycle changes in patients may include an unstable stance limb, insufficient foot clearance, inappropriate position of the foot, and inadequate step length.

Other neuromuscular diseases include genetic or syndromic conditions. Gait patterns can be quite variable and can be static or progressive. In certain disease processes weakness may be the main presenting symptom. Examples of these diseases are spinal muscular atrophy type I, congenital myotonic dystrophy,

Table 3 Septic arthritis versus transient synovitis		
	Septic Arthritis	**Transient Synovitis**
Temperature	>101.3°F	Low-grade fever
Ambulation	No	Limp
WBC	>12,000/μL	Normal-slight elevation
ESR	>40 mm/h	Normal-slight elevation
CRP	>2.5 mg/L	Normal-slight elevation
Joint fluid		
WBC	>50,000/μL	5000–15,000/μL
Polymorphonuclear leukocytes (PMNs)	>75%	Low
Gram stain	Positive *Staphylococcus aureus, Staphylococcus pneumoniae*, group B S treptococcus, *Kingella kingae*	Negative

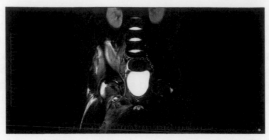

Fig. 13. Septic arthritis and osteomyelitis of the proximal femur on MRI in a 13-year-old. Imaging revealed fluid in the hip joint and edema of surrounding soft tissues in a patient who had complained of pain and difficulty walking. Plain radiographs were normal.

Duchenne muscular dystrophy, Charcot-Marie-Tooth, and Becker muscular dystrophy. Weakness usually progresses from proximal to distal.

History may be key in helping identify these patients. A child not walking by 18 months needs a further investigation.[40] During the examination, assessment for weakness will rely on functional examination, as they may not understand manual muscle testing. Have the child walk and jog in the hallway, and if stairs are available watch them go up and down. Ask the child to sit on the ground and watch them stand up. Gower sign indicates proximal muscle weakness, and the child will need to place their hands on, the lower extremities, essentially, climbing up the lower extremities with their upper extremities to stand.

Rheumatology
The most common rheumatologic diagnosis in children is juvenile inflammatory arthritis (JIA).[41] This autoimmune disease presents with joint pain and swelling. If a lower extremity is involved the child will often limp. Other systemic symptoms include morning stiffness, lethargy, recurrent fevers, rash, or loss of appetite. The diagnosis is often clinical, requiring at least 6 weeks of persistent joint swelling. Laboratory evaluation may reveal elevated systemic inflammatory markers (CRP or ESR); however, it may also be normal. An elevated ANA alone is *NOT* diagnostic of JIA but may be helpful in prognosis in the right clinical setting. An MRI with and without contrast may be considered in cases of persistent joint effusion if history or examination is not clear or consistent with acute injury or chronic effusion concerning for rheumatologic cause.

Genetic and metabolic
Duchene muscular dystrophy presents in boys 2 to 6 years old. Progressive weakness leads to gait abnormalities. Calf pseudohypertrophy is seen on physical examination. These patients also have a positive Gower sign. Other genetic conditions that can affect gait include hip instability associated with Down syndrome and general joint laxity associated with connective tissue disorders such as Ehlers-Danlos syndrome.

Rickets leads to poor calcification of the bones and can present as bowing of the lower limbs. The different forms include nutritional (vitamin D deficient), familial hypophosphatemic (vitamin D resistant), vitamin D dependent, hypophosphatasia, and renal osteodystrophy. Medical management may be sufficient for treatment of mild deformities.

Malignancy
Although relatively rare, malignancy can present as a gait change in children. Primary musculoskeletal tumors arise from the bone or soft tissue and are usually benign. They are often found incidentally after minor trauma. The most common benign tumors

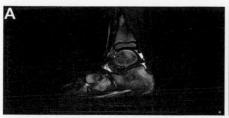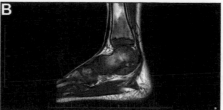

Fig. 14. A 9-year-old presented with difficulty walking and running 2 months after an "ankle sprain." Plain radiographs were normal. Sagittal MRI images of the ankle revealed pronounced marrow edema in the distal fibula; tibia; talus; calcaneus; navicular; cuboid; cuneiforms; and first, second, and fourth metatarsals. After additional workup he was diagnosed with pre-B acute lymphoblastic leukemia.

include osteochondroma, nonossifying fibroma, osteoid osteoma, aneurysmal bone cyst, unicameral or simple bone cyst, and Langerhans cell histiocytosis. Malignant bone tumors are the seventh most common childhood tumor.[17] Most are osteosarcomas and Ewing sarcomas. These cases usually present as pain and swelling in adolescents. Acute lymphocytic leukemia should be considered in patients with musculoskeletal pain including pain at night, a low WBC, and normal to low platelets in early presentation or overt pancytopenia[42] (**Fig. 14**).

SUMMARY

Pediatric gait changes may be normal variations or reveal concerning medical conditions. The primary care provider should have a good knowledge of age-appropriate findings, confidence with the lower extremity physical examination, and a wide differential diagnosis for these presentations. Reassuring patients and families of normal variations can limit unnecessary testing and stress, whereas prompt referral for urgent orthopedic conditions can limit morbidity and even mortality in pediatric patients.

CLINICS CARE POINTS

- Gait patterns consist of a combination of skeletal alignment and neuromuscular development.

- A normal gait pattern requires a normal functioning motor cortex, functioning skeleton, muscles and tendons, and skeletal alignment within appropriate range of function.

- A mature gait pattern typically presents in a more organized fashion around 7 to 8 years of age.

- Close to 50% of new referrals to pediatric orthopedic clinics are for children with normal variations in the lower extremities; as such, developing an understanding for the normal variation in skeletal development is important.

- Assessing gait can be overwhelming, as there is large variability due to numerous different causes for various gait patterns. Taking a good history and completing a thorough physical examination, assessing for symmetry, range of motion and flexibility, and pain, can help to narrow the differential diagnosis.

ACKNOWLEDGMENTS

James Weihe, MD and Gwen Sprague, MLS.

DISCLOSURE

The authors have nothing to disclose.

SUPPLEMENTARY DATA

Supplementary data related to this article can be found online at https://doi.org/10.1016/j.pop.2021.04.004.

REFERENCES

1. Sutherland DH, Olshen R, Cooper L, et al. The development of mature gait. J Bone Joint Surg Am 1980;62(3):336–53.
2. Dabney KW, Miller F. Cerebral Palsy. In: Abel M, editor. Orthopaedic knowledge update pediatrics 3. Rosemont (IL): American Academy of Orthopedic Surgeons; 2006. p. 94.
3. Kliegman RM. Nelson textbook of pediatrics. 21st edition. Elsevier; 2019.
4. Kotwick JE. Biomechanics of the foot and ankle. Clin Sports Med 1982;1(1): 19–34.
5. Rerucha CM, Dickison C, Baird DC. Lower Extremity Abnormalities in Children. Am Fam Physician 2017;96(4):226–33.
6. Scharf RJ, Scharf GJ, Stroustrup A. Developmental Milestones. Pediatr Rev 2016; 37(1):25–37 [quiz: 38, 47]. [Erratum in: Pediatr Rev. 2016;37(6):266].
7. Wilson CH. The musculoskeletal examination. In: Walker HK, Hall WD, Hurst JW, editors. Clinical methods: the history, physical, and laboratory examinations. 3rd edition. Boston: Butterworths; 1990. p. 767–8. Chapter 164.
8. Benard MA. Pediatric Considerations. Clin Podiatric Med Surg 2020;37(1): 125–50.
9. Lincoln TL, Suen PW. Common rotational variations in children. J Am Acad Orthop Surg 2003;11(5):312–20.
10. Staheli L. Rotational Problems in Children. J Bone Joint Surg 1993;75(6):939–49.
11. Wall EJ. Practical primary pediatric orthopedics. Nurs Clin North Am 2000;35(1): 95–113.
12. Carr JB, Yang S, Lather LA. Pediatric Pes Planus: A State-of-the-Art Review. Pediatrics 2016;137(3):e20151230.
13. Roach KE, Miles TP. Normal hip and knee active range of motion: the relationship to age. Phys Ther 1991 Sep;71(9):656–65. https://doi.org/10.1093/ptj/71.9.656. PMID: 1881956.
14. Diab M, Staheli L. Chapter 6 Foot and Ankle. In: Brian Brown, editor. Practice of paediatric orthopaedics. 3rd edition. Philadelphia: Lippincott Williams & Wilkins; 2016. p. 358–64.
15. Naqvi U, Sherman AI. Muscle Strength Grading. In: StatPearls. Treasure Island (FL): StatPearls Publishing; 2020. Available at: https://www.ncbi.nlm.nih.gov/books/NBK436008/.
16. Dolitsky R, DePaola K, Fernicola J, et al. Pediatric Musculoskeletal Infections. Pediatr Clin North Am 2020;67(1):59–69.
17. Singla A, Geller DS. Musculoskeletal Tumors. Pediatr Clin North Am 2020;67(1): 227–45.
18. Molony D, Hefferman G, Dodds M, et al. Normal variants in the paediatric orthopaedic population. Ir Med J 2006;99(1):13–4.
19. Jones S, Khandekar S, Tolessa E. Normal variants of the lower limbs in pediatric orthopedics. Intern J Clin Med 2013;4:12–7.

20. Greene WB. Genu varum and genu valgum in children: differential diagnosis and guidelines for evaluation. Compr Ther 1996;22(1):22–9.
21. Davids JR, Blackhurst DW, Allen BL. Radiographic evaluation of bowed legs in children. J Pediatr Orthop 2001;21(2):257–63.
22. Katz K, David R, Soudry M. Below-knee plaster cast for the treatment of metatarsus adductus. J Pediatr Orthop 1999;19(1):49–50.
23. Staheli LT. Torsion–treatment indications. Clin Orthop Relat Res 1989;247:61–6.
24. Heath CH, Staheli LT. Normal limits of knee angle in white children–genu varum and genu valgum. J Pediatr Orthop 1993;13(2):259–62.
25. Walker JL, Hosseinzadeh P, White H, et al. Idiopathic genu valgum and its association with obesity in children and adolescents. J Pediatr Orthop 2019;39(7): 347–52.
26. Khamis S, Carmeli E. Relationship and significance of gait deviations associated with limb length discrepancy: A systematic review. Gait & Posture 2017;57: 115–23.
27. Whitaker AT, Vuillermin C. Lower extremity growth and deformity. Curr Rev Musculoskelet Med 2016;9(4):454–61.
28. Morozova OM, Chang TF, Brown ME. Toe walking: when do we need to worry? Curr Probl Pediatr Adolesc Health Care 2017;47(7):156–60.
29. Payares-Lizano M, Pino C. Pediatric orthopedic examination. Pediatr Clin North Am 2020;67(1):1–21.
30. Herman MJ, Martinek M. The limping child. Pediatr Rev 2015;36(5):184–95 [quiz: 196–7].
31. Peck DM, Voss LM, Voss TT. Slipped capital femoral epiphysis: diagnosis and management. Am Fam Physician 2017;95(12):779–84.
32. Hosseinzadeh P, Hayes CB. Compartment Syndrome in Children. Orthop Clin North Am 2016;47(3):579–87.
33. Tenenbein M, Reed MH, Black GB. The toddler's fracture revisited. Am J Emerg Med 1990;8(3):208–11.
34. Singhal R, Perry DC, Khan FN, et al. The use of CRP within a clinical prediction algorithm for the differentiation of septic arthritis and transient synovitis in children. J Bone Joint Surg Br 2011;93(11):1556–61.
35. Vaquero-Picado A, González-Morán G, Garay EG, et al. Developmental dysplasia of the hip: update of management. EFORT Open Rev 2019;4(9):548–56.
36. Cook PC. Transient synovitis, septic hip, and Legg-Calvé-Perthes disease: an approach to the correct diagnosis. Pediatr Clin North Am 2014;61(6):1109–18.
37. Kim HK. Legg-Calvé-Perthes disease. J Am Acad Orthop Surg 2010;18(11): 676–86.
38. Fischer SU, Beattie TF. The limping child: epidemiology, assessment and outcome. J Bone Joint Surg Br 1999;81(6):1029–34.
39. Michel C, Collins C. Pediatric Neuromuscular Disorders. Pediatr Clin North Am 2020;67(1):45–57.
40. WHO Multicentre Growth Reference Study Group. WHO Motor Development Study: windows of achievement for six gross motor development milestones. Acta Paediatr Suppl 2006;450:86–95.
41. Palman J, Shoop-Worrall S, Hyrich K, et al. Update on the epidemiology, risk factors and disease outcomes of Juvenile idiopathic arthritis. Best Pract Res Clin Rheumatol 2018;32(2):206–22.
42. Jones OY, Spencer CH, Bowyer SL, et al. A multicenter case-control study on predictive factors distinguishing childhood leukemia from juvenile rheumatoid arthritis. Pediatrics 2006;117(5):e840–4.

Common Pediatric Musculoskeletal Issues

Brittney M. Richardson, MD, CAQSM[a],*, Meghane E. Masquelin, DO[b]

KEYWORDS

- Pediatric • Musculoskeletal • Imaging • Therapies • Physeal injury
- Apophyseal injury • Back pain

KEY POINTS

- More than 60 million children participate in organized sports, with more than half of them participating in more than 1 sport.
- Because of the volume of young athletes, the rate at which there are overuse and acute injuries is significant.
- Physical therapy is often helpful in addressing the muscular imbalances commonly encountered in amateur athletes.
- Although it often does not change the medical management, advanced imaging can help solidify diagnosis and predict the time to return to play.
- Although back pain is often self-limited in pediatric patients, prolonged symptoms should be investigated.

INTRODUCTION

Children are some of the most resilient humans on earth. Although they may present with significant disorders, musculoskeletal and otherwise, this resilience allows them to persevere while attempting to maintain their high spirits and playfulness. Throughout this article, many of the musculoskeletal issues children can develop are highlighted and presentation, diagnosis, treatment, and prognosis are discussed to assist in early diagnosis and treatment of this group and transition back to normal activity. This article addresses common injuries and disorders seen in the active pediatric population.

Participating in sports is one of the prized pastimes in the United States. Nearly 60 million children participate in organized sports, with about half participating in multiple sports. That number is growing and results in nearly 2 million injuries annually among high school athletes in America.[1] Although there are benefits of physical activity, including decreasing risk of obesity, improving cardiovascular fitness, and

[a] Department of Family and Geriatric Medicine, University of Louisville School of Medicine, 215 Central Avenue, Suite 205, Louisville, KY 40208, USA; [b] University of Louisville Family Medicine Residency Program, 201 Abraham Flexner Way, Suite 690, Louisville, KY 40202, USA
* Corresponding author.
E-mail address: brittney.richardson@louisville.edu

interpersonal development, this comes with the risk of injury.[2] At this level of participation, the likelihood of injury is significant.[1,3]

PHYSEAL INJURIES

The physis, also called epiphyseal plate, physeal plate, or growth plate, is a cartilaginous disc in the skeletally immature separating the epiphysis from the metaphysis in long bones. Made up of hyaline cartilage, it is responsible for the longitudinal growth of bone by the process of chondrocyte proliferation.[4] Over time, the growth plate disappears and is replaced by bone formed by osteoblasts cells through ossification. The lack of calcification in this area of bone makes it susceptible to injuries because of its inability to counterattack shearing stress. Injuries of the growth plate, or physeal injuries, make up 15% to 30% of all bony injuries in children.[5]

Little League Shoulder

Little league shoulder is an injury of the proximal humerus at the physeal plate. More specifically, it is a Salter-Harris I or epiphysiolysis fracture, often seen in skeletally immature overhead-throwing athletes.[5] The Salter-Harris classification (**Table 1**) is used to categorize fractures at the physeal plate through the zone of provisional calcification, a layer of noncalcified bone that is consequently weak and more susceptible to injury.[6] This injury is related to repetitive torsion and distraction stresses at the physis causing widening of the epiphyseal plate and resulting in significant pain. The development of this injury results from increased frequency and volume of pitches seen in young boys participating in Little League baseball.[1]

Presentation:

- Overhead athlete, age 11 to 16 years, typically a pitcher, with shoulder pain[5]
- Decreased velocity and control of throws
- Pain is worse at the end of the pitch
- Pain improves with rest
- Pitching daily without rest
- No acute injury

The physical examination usually reveals normal range of motion with tenderness of the proximal lateral humerus.[5] In particular, the shoulder examination may show

Table 1	
Salter-Harris classification of physeal injuries	
Salter-Harris Classification	**Description**
Type I	Transverse fracture through the growth plate separating the epiphysis from the metaphysis
Type II	Transverse fracture through the growth plate with an oblique fracture through the metaphysis
Type III	Transverse fracture through the growth plate with a vertical fracture through the epiphysis
Type IV	Vertical fracture through the metaphysis, physis, and epiphysis
Type V	Compression fracture of the growth plate

Data from Cepela, DJ, Tartaglione, JP, Dooley, TP, Patel, PN. Classifications In Brief: Salter-Harris Classification of Pediatric Physeal Fractures. *Clinical Orthopedics and Related Research.* 2016;474:2531-2537.

decreased strength with external rotation and abduction, as well as pain with resisted internal and external rotation. On examination of the scapulae, there is often evidence of atrophy leading to scapular dyskinesia caused by poor scapular stabilization and imbalance of muscle strength.[5]

Radiographs of bilateral shoulders with internal and external rotation views provide good visualization of the bilateral humeral physeal plates. Widening of one side compared with the other confirms the diagnosis (**Fig. 1**).[5]

Treatment:

- Rest
- Physical therapy
  - Core strengthening
  - Scapular stabilization
  - Posterior capsule stretching
  - Rotator cuff strengthening
  - Throwing mechanics
- No throwing until pain resolves
- Gradual return to throwing after 3-month period of rest[5]

Prevention of Little League shoulder involves following strict activity-related guidelines.[5] Athletes should avoid pitching breaking balls until skeletally mature and should follow pitch count guidelines based on age.[7] Working on maintaining good throwing mechanics and core strength are the most important factors in preventing injuries.[5] Because of early sport specialization often leading to overuse injuries, avoiding year-round pitching is also a good preventive measure.

APOPHYSEAL INJURIES

The apophysis is a normal developmental outgrowth of bone found where major tendons and ligaments attach. It arises from an ossification center separate from the

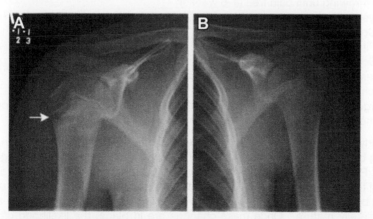

Fig. 1. Chronic right proximal humeral physeal stress fracture (Little League shoulder) in a 14-year-old right-hand-dominant pitcher. (*A*) Anteroposterior [AP] radiograph of the affected right shoulder shows abnormal widening and marginal irregularity of the lateral aspect of the growth plate(*arrow*). (*B*) AP comparison radiograph of the unaffected left shoulder shows normal width and well-defined margins of the intact physis. (*From* Lomasney LM, Lim-Dunham JE, Cappello T, Annes J. Imaging of the pediatric athlete: use and overuse. Radiol Clin North Am. 2013 Mar;51(2):215-26; with permission.)

mother bone that fuses later in development.[8] There is usually no direct articulation with another bone or joint. Until completely fused, it can easily be injured during repetitive activities because of shear stress applied to it by attached tendons and ligaments. These injuries account for up to 16% of all sport-related injuries.[8]

Little League Elbow

Little League elbow is an apophyseal injury to the medial elbow seen in skeletally immature throwing athletes.[1] Inflammation of the apophysis results from repetitive microtrauma from valgus stress overloading medial structures and leading to pain. This condition develops from increased volume and frequency of throws, with pain more pronounced during the late cocking and early acceleration phases of throwing mechanics.[1]

Presentation:

- Throwing athletes, usually a pitcher, aged 9 to 14 years
- Decreased velocity and/or accuracy of throws
- Medial elbow pain that improves with rest[9]
- No acute injury

On physical examination, there is tenderness to palpation at the medial epicondyle and pain without laxity with valgus stress of the elbow.[9] As in Little League shoulder, there is often a correlation with decreased core strength and scapular stabilization resulting in increased stress isolated to the elbow during throwing.

This injury can be seen on anteroposterior and lateral radiographs of the elbow, where evidence of apophyseal widening can be observed compared with the contralateral side (**Fig. 2**).[9] There may also be fragmentations or avulsions of the medial elbow. MRI is a beneficial additional imaging technique in cases where there is concern for laxity of the elbow with valgus stress because MRI shows the ulnar collateral ligament in detail.[1]

Treatment:

- No throwing until pain free (4–6 weeks)[9]
- Physical therapy
  o Core strengthening
  o Pitching mechanics
  o Scapular stabilization
- Nonsteroidal antiinflammatory medication and ice[9]
- Pitch count compliance
- Surgery, using open reduction and internal fixation, is indicated if the apophysis is more than 5 mm from the distal humerus[9]

Similarly to Little League shoulder, prevention of Little League elbow lies in limiting throwing by following the appropriate pitch count guidelines based on the age of the patient.[1] Proper rest between practice and games as well as development of accurate throwing technique are key. Curve balls and sliders put a significant amount of stress on the elbow, having an 86% increase in risk for elbow pain, and should be avoided until skeletally mature.[1] Once these changes are in place, the likelihood of reinjury because of increased stress at the apophysis is decreased.

Osgood-Schlatter Syndrome and Sinding-Larson-Johansson Syndrome

Apophyseal injury at the knee can present in 2 ways: traction apophysitis at the tibial tuberosity or a similar mechanism at lower pole of the patella. Osgood-Schlatter syndrome occurs secondary to forceful contraction of the quadriceps tendon in the

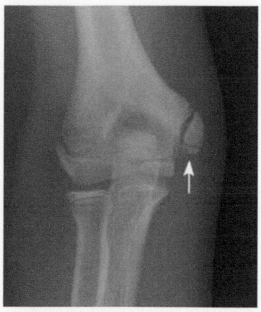

Fig. 2. Chronic medial epicondyle apophysitis and physeal injury secondary to valgus stress (Little League elbow) in a 13-year-old right-hand-dominant baseball player. AP radiograph of the right elbow shows abnormal fragmentation of the medial epicondyle (*arrow*) with excessive widening, irregularity, and sclerosis of the adjacent growth plate. (*From* Lomasney LM, Lim-Dunham JE, Cappello T, Annes J. Imaging of the pediatric athlete: use and overuse. Radiol Clin North Am. 2013 Mar;51(2):215-26; with permission.)

extensor mechanism of the knee seen in repetitive jumping.[10] It is often seen in adolescent basketball and volleyball athletes and leads to pain at the tibial tuberosity. Interestingly, it is only found bilaterally in about 20% to 30% of patients.[10]

Presentation:

- Pain at the anterior knee exacerbated by kneeling and jumping[1]
- Jumping athlete (basketball, volleyball, track and field)[10]
- Boys aged 12 to 15 years or girls aged 8 to 12 years[10]
- No acute injury

The examination normally reveals tenderness to palpation at the tibial tubercle and pain with resisted knee extension. There is often evidence of swelling or enlargement of the tibial tuberosity.[10] Diagnosis is confirmed with examination and imaging of the knee. Frequently, there is irregularity or even fragmentation of the tubercle on lateral radiographs of the knee (**Fig. 3**).[11] An MRI scan is not necessary for diagnosis, but possible findings include soft tissue swelling of the structures surrounding the patellar tendon at the insertion on the tibia, and thickening and edema of the inferior patellar tendon.[10]

Treatment:

- Conservative options:
  - Rest, cryotherapy, activity modification, and nonsteroidal antiinflammatory drugs
  - Physical therapy aimed at core strengthening and quadriceps stretching
  - Straps, sleeves, or taping to decrease tension on the apophysitis

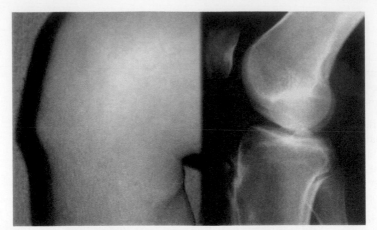

Fig. 3. Osgood-Schlatter disease. (*From* Waldman, SD. Chapter 116: Osgood-Schlatter Disease *Atlas of Common Pain Syndromes*, Fourth Edition. Elsevier, Inc.; 2019:459-463; with permission.)

- ○ 90% of patients have complete resolution
- ○ Cast immobilization for 6 weeks for severe symptoms[10]
- Operative management
  - ○ Ossicle excision in refractory cases, which occur 10% of the time[10]
  - ○ Patients must fail conservative therapy

In Sinding-Larsen-Johansson syndrome, there is development of anterior knee pain at the inferior patella caused by traction of the patellar tendon resulting in apophyseal plate inflammation. This apophyseal inflammation occurs at the inferior pole of the patella at the proximal patellar tendon attachment causing traction apophysitis.[1] The presentation of this injury is very similar to Osgood-Schlatter disease with the exception of patients being slightly younger, generally around the age of 10 to 14 years.[12] Diagnosis is mostly clinical and is often achieved without imaging. If radiographs are obtained, spurring can be visualized in chronic cases. Furthermore, they can also be seen on MRI T1 sagittal views. Bony edema is noticeable on MRI T2 sagittal views.[1,12] Treatment is largely conservative because the condition is often self-limiting.[12]

Sever Disease

Sever disease is the most common cause of heel pain in skeletally immature athletes, resulting from an overuse injury at the calcaneal apophysis. It is frequently seen around the time of a growth spurt in a running or jumping athlete.[1] The apophysitis develops secondary to the significant force experienced at the heel during the heel strike phase of normal gait in conjunction with the traction stress created by the gastrosoleus complex.[13]

Presentation:

- Age 9 to 12 years, more commonly male than female
- Heel pain exacerbated by activity and heel strike
- No acute injury

On examination, the full range of motion of the ankle is preserved but there are tight heel cords palpable along the Achilles tendon without significant tenderness or defect.[13] Pain is elicited with a calcaneal squeeze test involving medial-lateral compression over the calcaneal tuberosity.[13] In addition, there is tenderness to palpation over the calcaneal apophysis with pain on single-leg hop, which exaggerates repetitive heel strikes. A radiograph is initially not necessary with most classic presentations. If a radiograph is obtained, it may show widening, sclerosis, or fragmentation of the calcaneal apophysis (**Fig. 4**).[1,13]

Treatment:

- Achilles tendon stretches
- Rest, cryotherapy, nonsteroidal antiinflammatory drugs
- Activity modification
- Use of heel cups or heel pads
- Immobilization in short-leg cast or controlled ankle motion (CAM) walking boot for refractory pain

Recurrence is common but symptoms are self-limited and ultimately resolve with skeletal maturity and closure of the apophysis.[1] There is no role for operative management in recurrent cases. Prevention involves altering activity as necessary to avoid exacerbation.

Apophyseal Avulsion Fractures

The pelvis is susceptible to avulsion injuries at various apophyseal plates, resulting in separating of the apophysis from the body of the pelvis or femur. In skeletally immature patients, sudden forceful muscle contraction causes stress at the weakest area of bone. The same mechanism is likely to result in a muscle strain or tendon injury in skeletally mature patients. Common activities leading to this subset of injuries are kicking, jumping, and sprinting, which are fundamentals to many sports, including rugby, track, soccer, ice hockey, and gymnastics.[14] These injuries occur most frequently at the ischial tuberosity, where the hamstrings (semitendinosus, biceps femoris, and semimembranosus), the anterior superior iliac spine (origination of the sartorius), and the anterior inferior iliac spine (rectus femoris) originate.[14] There are numerous sites of possible injuries in the pelvis, which are listed in **Table 2**.[14]

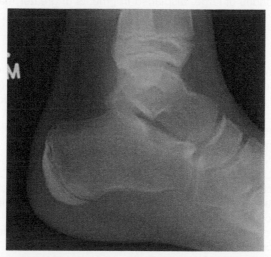

Fig. 4. Calcaneal apophysis. (*From* Hoang QB, Mortazavi M. Pediatric overuse injuries in sports. Adv Pediatr. 2012;59(1):359-83; with permission.)

Table 2
Pelvic apophyses-muscle attachments and ages at time of their ossification

Apophysis	Originating Muscle	Inserting Muscle	Age of Appearance (y)	Age of Closure (y)
Greater trochanter	None	Gluteus maximus and medius, external hip rotators	9–10	14–16
Lesser trochanter	None	Iliopsoas	9–10	14–16
Anterior superior iliac spine	Sartorius	None	12–14	14–16
Anterior inferior iliac spine	Rectus femoris	None	12–14	14–16
Iliac crest	Tensor fasciae latae	Internal and external obliques, transversus abdominis	13–15	16–18
Ischial tuberosity	Biceps femoris, hip extensors	None	15–17	21–25

From Hoang QB, Mortazavi M. Pediatric overuse injuries in sports. Adv Pediatr. 2012;59(1):359-83; with permission.

Presentation:

- Teenage boy or girl with acute pain during strenuous activity
- Usually hear or feel a pop, which is immediately followed by pain[1]
- Weight bearing causes pain
- Pain with palpation and passive stretching of muscle and tendon
- Radiograph (anteroposterior pelvis) confirms clinical suspicion

Treatment involves rest, ice, and no to partial weight bearing depending on the severity of pain. Gradual return to play can be initiated after pain has subsided and strength has been regained. Very rarely is any surgical intervention required; it is reserved for incidences of large, displaced fragments of greater than 2 cm from the pelvis or femur.

BACK PAIN

Back pain in children and young adults most often represents as a benign self-limited entity. However, persistent or worsening pain could be a sign of potentially significant abnormalities and should be properly investigated. This presentation could be secondary to inflammation, infection, neoplasm, or congenital causes. A timely evaluation is paramount to prevent further progression of the underlying cause, to initiate appropriate management, and to avoid complications.

Scoliosis

Scoliosis is a structural alternation of the spine that is defined as a lateral curvature of the vertebrae greater than 10°. The most common cause of scoliosis is idiopathic (80% of cases); however, it may be associated with neuromuscular conditions, skeletal dysplasia, or congenital spinal deformity.[15] Scoliosis is classified as early onset when diagnosed before the age of 10 years.[15]

Scoliosis is often diagnosed by primary care physicians. Although the United States Preventive Services Task Force (USPSTF) has determined that it is no longer beneficial to screen adolescents between the ages of 10 and 18 years for scoliosis, it is important to remember that this only applies to asymptomatic patients and does not apply to children or adolescents who present with back pain, breathing difficulties, abnormal imaging studies, or obvious deformity in spinal curvature.[16] Alternatively, the American Academy of Orthopedic Surgeons, the Scoliosis Research Society, the Pediatric Orthopedic Society of North America, and the American Academy of Pediatrics all advocate screening for scoliosis in girls at 10 and 12 years of age and once in adolescent boys at 13 or 14 years of age.[17] The Adam forward bend test and scoliometers are the 2 most useful clinical screening methods for the early detection of scoliosis.[15] Confirmation of diagnosis and further severity classification is achieved with imaging and by measuring the Cobb angle (**Fig. 5**).[18,19] The size of the angle, and thus the degree of severity, is used to identify the next step in management, including physical therapy, bracing, and/or surgery.

Spondylolysis

Spondylolysis is a unilateral or bilateral, acute or chronic fracture of the pars interarticularis. It is secondary to repetitive microtrauma and hyperextension of the developing

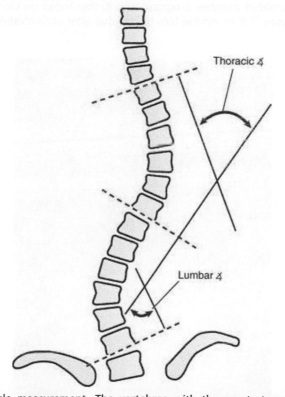

Thoracic ∡

Lumbar ∡

Fig. 5. Cobb angle measurement. The vertebrae with the greatest amount of tilt are selected as the end vertebrae. Lines are drawn perpendicular to the end plates of the vertebrae. The angle formed at the intersection of these lines is the Cobb angle. If a second curve is present below the primary curve, the original curve's lower vertebra becomes the top vertebra when measuring the second curve, and the same line along its surface is used. (*From* Stephens Richards, B, Sucato, DJ, Johnston, CE. Chapter 12: Scoliosis. *Pediatric Orthopaedics,* Fifth Edition. Saunders/Elsevier, Inc.; 2014:206-307; with permission.)

spine. It is the most common cause of low back pain with reproducible point tenderness in children more than 10 years old. In addition, it is more common in boys than in girls and most (85%–95%) defects occur at the L5 vertebral level.[15] The repetitive extension and twisting motions of the lumbar spine seen in soccer, football, gymnastics, and volleyball are the reasons why these sports are most commonly associated with this type of injury..[20] If spondylolysis is not identified and managed in a timely fashion, continued biomechanical stress can progress to spondylolisthesis, the anterior displacement of the fractured vertebral body, and cause neurologic symptoms secondary to spinal canal or neural foramina stenosis.

The gold standard for diagnosing spondylolysis or spondylolisthesis is with posteroanterior, lateral, and oblique upright radiographs of the lumbar spine (**Fig. 6**).[20–22] The oblique view shows a focal bandlike lucency with adjacent sclerosis or elongation of the pars interarticularis, which is often referred to as the Scotty dog sign. Other more advanced imaging techniques, such as computed tomography scan and MRI, can be used to confirm the diagnosis by detecting bony edema, which is often missed on plain radiographs..[20] Once diagnosed, conservative treatment options include the discontinuation of sporting activity and a combination of stabilization and physical therapy. This approach specifically entails using a full-time Boston brace for 8 to 12 weeks, a graduated exercise program, and further focus on isometric core and hamstring exercises.[20] If an athlete fails to improve after conservative management,

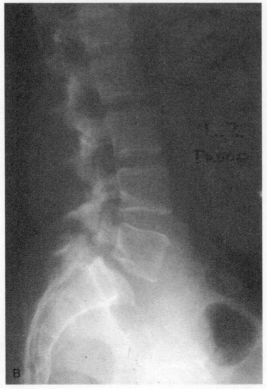

Fig. 6. Lateral radiograph of an L5 to S1 spondylolisthesis. (*From* Nolte, MT, DeWald, CJ. Chapter 116: Spondylolysis and Spondylolisthesis. *Essential Orthopaedics*, Second Edition. Elsevier, Inc.; 2020:461-467; with permission.)

surgery should be considered. Additional surgical criteria include inability to return to play after more than 6 months and worsening imaging studies.[20] For athletes with spondylolisthesis, pars repair and debridement of the fibrous defect may be the preferred surgical intervention. If disc degeneration was previous appreciated on imaging, then anterior and/or posterior fusion may be required instead.[20] Regarding the recovery process, athletes should expect to return to sport after 6 to 12 months unless a lumbar fusion was performed, which could be a career-ending intervention because return to contact sports is rarely recommended by physicians after that.[20] With a timely conservative treatment plan, surgical intervention is seldom necessary and most young athletes are expected to make a full return to play.[23]

CLINICS CARE POINTS

- Because children are participating in organized sports at an increased rate, the incidence of overuse injuries is increasing.

- Deriving a complete history is important in revealing unhealthy levels of activity in the skeletally immature and details of acute injuries.

- The mainstays of treatment of physeal, apophyseal, and back injuries are activity modification, physical therapy, nonsteroidal antiinflammatory medicines, cryotherapy, and identifying potential flaws in mechanics or frequency of activity.

- Plain radiograph is often helpful, especially when compared with the other side, in the instance of apophyseal injuries, to aid in obtaining a diagnosis.

- Operative management is often reserved for refractory cases and special instances, such as the injuries discussed in this article.

- Although encouragement to be active in adolescence is important for social development, cardiovascular fitness, and decreased risk of obesity, it is equally significant to educate patients and families about the need to monitor activity level and risk of overuse injuries.

DISCLOSURE

The authors have nothing to disclose.

REFERENCES

1. Lomasney LM, Lim-Dunham JE, Cappello T, et al. Imaging of the pediatric athlete: use and overuse. Radiol Clin North Am 2013;51(2):215–26.
2. Logan K, Cuff S. AAP council on sports medicine and fitness. Organized sports for children, preadolescents, and adolescents. Pediatrics 2019;143(6): e20190997.
3. Mariscalco MW, Saluan P. Upper extremity injuries in the adolescent athlete. Sports Med Arthrosc Rev 2011;19(1):17–26.
4. Enishi T, Matsuura T, Suzue N, et al. Cartilage degeneration at symptomatic persistent olecranon physis in adolescent baseball players. Adv Orthop 2014; 2014:545438.
5. Osbahr DC, Kim HJ, Dugas JR. Little league shoulder. Curr Opin Pediatr 2010; 22(1):35–40.
6. Cepela DJ, Tartaglione JP, Dooley TP, et al. Classifications in brief: salter-harris classification of pediatric physeal fractures. Clin Orthop Relat Res 2016;474: 2531–7.

7. Lyman S, Fleisig GS, Andrews JR, et al. Effect of pitch type, pitch count, and pitching mechanics on risk of elbow and shoulder pain in youth baseball pitchers. Am J Sports Med 2002;30(4):463–8.

8. Longo UG, Ciuffreda M, Locher J, et al. Apophyseal injuries in children's and youth sports. Br Med Bull 2016;120(Issue 1):139–59.

9. Klingele KE, Kocher MS. Little league elbow: valgus overload injury in the paediatric athlete. Sports Med 2002;32(15):1005–15.

10. Kujala UM, Kvist M, Heinonen O. Osgood-Schlatter's disease in adolescent athletes: Retrospective study of incidence and duration. Am J Sports Med 1985; 13(4):236–41.

11. Waldman SD. Chapter 116: osgood-schlatter disease *Atlas of common pain syndromes*. 4th edition. Philadelphia, PA: Elsevier, Inc; 2019. p. 459–63.

12. Kuehnast M, Mahomed N, Mistry B. Sinding-Larsen-Johansson syndrome. South Afr J Child Health 2012;6(3):90–2.

13. Ramponi D. Sever's disease (Calcaneal Apophysitis). Adv Emerg Nurs J 2019; 41(1):10–4.

14. Hoang QB, Mortazavi M. Pediatric overuse injuries in sports. Adv Pediatr 2012; 56(1):359–83.

15. Calloni SF, Huisman TA, Poretti A, et al. Back pain and scoliosis in children: when to image, what to consider. Neuroradiol J 2017;30(5):393–404.

16. US Preventative Task Force. Screening for Adolescent Idiopathic Scoliosis US Preventive Services Task Force Recommendation Statement. JAMA 2018; 319(2):165–72.

17. Hresko MT, Talwakar VR, Schwend RM. SRS/POSNA/AAOS/AAP position statement: screening for the early detection for idiopathic scoliosis in adolescents. 2015. Available at: https://www.srs.org/about-srs/news-and-announcements/ position -statement—screening-for-the-early-detection-for -idiopathic-scoliosis-in-adolescents. Accessed November 14, 2020.

18. Goethem JV, Campenhourt AV, Hauwe L, et al. Scoliosis. Neuroimaging Clin North Am 2007;17(1):105–15.

19. Stephens Richards B, Sucato DJ, Johnston CE. Chapter 12: scoliosis. *Pediatric orthopaedics*. 5th edition. Philadelphia, PA: Saunders/Elsevier, Inc; 2014. p. 206–307.

20. Ball JR, Harris CB, Lee J, et al. Lumbar spine injuries in sports: review of the literature and current treatment recommendations. Sports Med Open 2019;5(1):26.

21. Wright J, Balaji V, Montgomery AS. Spondylosis and spondylolisthesis. Orthop Trauma 2013;27(4):195–200.

22. Nolte MT, DeWald CJ. Chapter 116: spondylolysis and spondylolisthesis. *Essential orthopaedics*. 2nd edition. Philadelphia, PA: Elsevier, Inc; 2020. p. 461–7.

23. Goetzinger S, Courtney S, Yee K, et al. Spondylolysis in young athletes: an overview emphasizing nonoperative management. J Sports Med 2020;2020:9235958.

Common Dental Issues in Pediatrics

Jeffrey M. Meyer, MD*, Nicole Bichir, MD, Sheridan Langford, MD

KEYWORDS

- Dental health • Caries • Teeth • Trauma • Children

KEY POINTS

- Dental disease is prevalent in childhood, and much of it can be prevented. Both medical and dental providers play a role in such prevention.
- Dental risk assessments should be used routinely at well child checks.
- Medical providers should endorse good dental hygiene and encourage the establishment of a dental home for children by 1 year of age.
- Fluoride treatments should be routinely offered at well child checkups, especially for children at high risk of caries.

INTRODUCTION

Dental health is an underrecognized component of comprehensive pediatric care. The mouth serves not only as the start of the alimentary canal and plays a critical role in nutrition but also functions in articulation, communication, and cosmesis. Dental disorders at any age can cause substantial functional deficits and negatively impact quality of life; pediatric dental problems can also set the stage for difficulties with lasting impacts into adulthood. In addition, pediatric dental health is complicated by the development of first the primary and then the permanent dentition. As such, pediatric health care providers must be prepared to evaluate a variety of dental conditions, provide education and preventative health interventions, and collaborate with dental providers to ensure quality outcomes through childhood and beyond.

General Dental Anatomy

Both primary and permanent teeth are composed of a 3-layer anatomic structure. First, there is a protective outer layer of enamel, which is the hard, highly mineralized layer. This layer is composed primarily of calcium and phosphate ions. Below the enamel is the softer layer of dentin. Dentin is yellowish in appearance and is sensitive when exposed by trauma or decay of the enamel. At the deepest layer of the tooth is

The authors have no commercial or financial conflicts of interest to disclose.
UofL Department of Pediatrics, 571 S. Floyd Street, Louisville, KY 40202, USA
* Corresponding author.
E-mail address: jeff.meyer@louisville.edu

the pulp, containing the neurovascular core of the tooth and functioning to continue dentin formation. Branches of the fifth cranial nerve provide the nervous supply to each tooth. The teeth are set in their sockets along the alveolar processes by periodontal ligaments. Each tooth receives its neurovascular supply from this anchor point deep into the apex of the root of the tooth.[1]

Primary dentition

Normal patterns of primary dental eruption can be variable in timing, but the average age of primary dental eruption is at 7 months, typically beginning with the lower central incisors. Dental eruption is usually symmetric. Infants often have the full complement of 8 central incisors by 12 months of age and all primary teeth by 3 years of age (**Table 1**).

Permanent dentition

The transition from primary to permanent teeth begins with the eruption of the first permanent molar at approximately 6 years of age. The process of exfoliation of the primary teeth and eruption of permanent teeth continues for approximately 6 years. The last teeth to erupt are the third permanent molars or "wisdom teeth" at around 19 years of age (**Fig. 1**, **Table 2**).

Oral Examination of the Newborn and Young Infant

Natal and neonatal teeth

Normal newborns are born without erupted dentition. However, 1 in 2000 newborns is born with teeth or experiences early tooth eruption in the neonatal period.[1] The term natal teeth refers to teeth present in the oral cavity at birth; neonatal teeth refer to teeth erupted within the first 30 days after birth. Ninety percent of natal or neonatal teeth are mandibular and a part of the normal primary dentition, rather than supernumerary.[2] Normal-appearing prematurely erupted teeth that are not causing significant feeding problems or soft tissue ulcerations should be retained. Supernumerary, abnormal-appearing, or loose teeth may need to be removed. Loose teeth can be a choking hazard.

Gingival cysts in the newborn

Gingival cysts are small inclusion cysts formed during embryologic development. These cysts are asymptomatic, do not grow, and usually disappear within weeks. Gingival cysts are named according to their location in the oral cavity and composition.

Table 1
Average age of eruption (in months) of the primary teeth

	Lower (Mandibular) Jaw	Upper (Maxillary) Jaw
Central incisor	7 mo	8 mo
Lateral incisor	8 mo	9 mo
Cuspid (canine)	17 mo	17 mo
First primary molar	13 mo	13 mo
Second primary molar	22 mo	22 mo

Data from Martin B. Oral Disorders. In: Zitelli BJ, McIntire SC, Nowalk AJ, eds. Oral Disorders Zitelli and Davis' atlas of pediatric physical diagnosis. 6th ed. Elsevier; 2018.

Tooth Identification

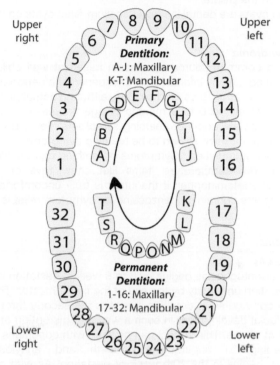

Fig. 1. Dental nomenclature for primary and permanent dentition.

Table 2
Average age of eruption (in years) of the permanent teeth

	Lower (Mandibular) Jaw	Upper (Maxillary) Jaw
Central incisor	7 y	8 y
Lateral incisor	8 y	9 y
Cuspid (canine)	10 y	11 y
First bicuspid	11 y	10 y
Second bicuspid	12 y	11 y
First permanent molar	6 y	6 y
Second permanent molar	12 y	12 y
Third permanent molar	19 y	19 y

Data from Martin B. Oral Disorders. In: Zitelli BJ, McIntire SC, Nowalk AJ, eds. *Oral Disorders Zitelli and Davis' atlas of pediatric physical diagnosis.* 6th ed. Elsevier; 2018.

- Epstein pearls are keratin-filled cysts on the midpalatine raphe.
- Bohn nodules are mucus gland cysts on the buccal or lingual aspect of the alveolar ridge or on the palate.
- Dental lamina cysts are dental lamina epithelium-filled cysts on the crest of alveolar ridge.[2]

Infant teething syndrome

Infant teething is a common source of concern raised at well child examinations. Around 4 months of age, many infants begin to experience a period of increased salivation and chewing on hands, toys, and so forth, although actual primary tooth eruption usually occurs closer to 6 to 9 months of age. Increased salivation, gingival irritation, and fussiness are common teething symptoms. Fever greater than 102°F and loose stools have not been shown to be teething symptoms, although these beliefs persist in many communities.[3] Symptoms of teething can be alleviated with the use of chilled or room-temperature items like chew toys or with a weight-appropriate dose of acetaminophen if the infant is truly uncomfortable. The use of numbing gels or creams containing benzocaine for symptom relief is not recommended for infants.[4]

Congenital Problems

Developmental issues

Primary dentition odontogenesis begins by 6 to 8 weeks' gestation in the embryonic stage, with calcification underway by the end of the first trimester. The first branchial arch of ectoderm contributes to dentition, whereas the second through sixth arches contribute to orofacial development in such a way that disruption of any part of this process can impact others. This impact can be seen with conditions such as cleft lip and palate leading to supernumerary teeth and ankylosis. Permanent dentition formation begins in the 20th week of gestation. As with other organ systems, odontogenesis can be affected by maternal factors, TORCH (toxoplasmosis, other agents, rubella, cytomegalovirus, herpes simplex) infections, teratogen exposures, and metabolic or genetic problems. Typically, the earlier in pregnancy these factors are present, the worse the outcome. Some permanent dentition continues to develop postnatally and can be affected by nutrition, chemotherapy, infection, mass effect, or trauma.

Infections

TORCH infections can lead to a broad range of birth defects including craniofacial anomalies, but some infections specifically affect odontogenesis. Cytomegalovirus can cause enamel hypoplasia.[5] Congenital rubella syndrome includes effects from growth restriction and can cause high palate and dental agenesis.[6] Congenital syphilis classically causes Hutchinson teeth (notched incisors), moon or bud molars, and mulberry molars among other pathognomonic findings.[7]

Teratogens

Teratogens include environmental chemicals, medications, illicit drugs, alcohol, and tobacco exposure, resulting in a variety of malformations. Fetal exposure to tetracyclines during the second and third trimesters can cause discoloration of the enamel of primary dentition; it is therefore recommended to avoid their use during pregnancy and even through early childhood. Antiepileptic drugs are also known to cause dental issues. Valproate conveys the highest risk of dental anomalies, especially in high-dose monotherapy or combination therapy with carbamazepine and other antiepileptics; this carries increased risk of facial dysmorphisms.[8,9]

Genetic or metabolic diseases

Genetic diseases cause an array of phenotypes, only some of which are well characterized. Compared with temporary disruptive factors as discussed previously, genetic conditions have a more global effect, involving both primary and permanent dentition. Specialized dental care is needed due to the high risk of caries and should be prioritized even amid complex medical problems. The most severe and well-known genetic disorders associated with abnormal dentition are as follows:

- Ectodermal dysplasia: collection of disorders of hair, skin, sweat glands, and teeth with hypodontia, cone-shaped teeth, or rarely anodontia.
- Amelogenesis imperfecta: autosomal dominant condition leading to hypoplasia or absence of the enamel with small, brown, misshapen teeth.
- Dentinogenesis imperfecta: autosomal dominant condition leading to hypoplasia of dentin with discolored, opalescent teeth. Type 1 is associated with osteogenesis imperfecta, whereas type 2 is more severe.[10]
- Both Down syndrome and Crouzon syndrome are associated with hypodontia.
- Ciliopathic genetic conditions such as primary ciliary dyskinesia or Bardet-Biedl syndrome cause heterogeneous dental developmental defects.[11]

Delayed eruption

If the first tooth has not erupted by 12 months of life, or if subsequent dentition is not erupting as expected, it is important to establish the presence of teeth. Referral to a pediatric dentist for panorex radiography is recommended. As panorex radiography is not performed at all radiology centers, calling to determine availability may be necessary.

An absent tooth can be acquired or due to agenesis. Agenesis is caused by disrupted development during odontogenesis, as triggered by exposure to maternal infection, certain drugs, or genetic diseases. Acquired absent dentition or damaged teeth are often caused by chemotherapy, infection, or trauma. Referral for genetic testing is recommended unless the absence is undoubtedly acquired. Treatment involves dental implants or prosthetics.

If a tooth is present, ankylosis, crowding from the persistent presence of primary teeth, or a mispositioned tooth may block eruption. Hyperdontia can exacerbate this problem by causing overcrowding and ankylosis, which can be painful. Dental referral for extraction or orthodontic care is necessary to treat and prevent malocclusion.[10]

Malocclusion and Crowding

Malocclusion is a common problem. Any disruption in development, from gross craniofacial anomalies to more indolent and common problems can lead to clinically significant malocclusion. Dental caries or infections leading to unilateral mastication can alter facial growth and impact developing permanent dentition due to the asymmetric pressure. Small stature or malnutrition can contribute to overcrowded teeth and asymmetric eruption.

Habits

Habits disrupting the normal position of teeth are both prevalent and treatable. Thumb sucking, tongue thrusting, and lip or cheek sucking are behaviors that most children outgrow between 2 and 4 years of age. Buy-in from the child is essential for treatment. Education and positive reinforcements like sticker charts can be useful first-line treatments. Persistent behaviors can also be deterred by physically blocking the hands with socks or gloves, plastic thumb shields, finger guards, or the application of a bitter substance on the involved digit or digits. If the behavior persists at the arrival of permanent dentition, refer to a dentist for the insertion of a mouth appliance (eg, palatal crib, lip guard).

Prolonged pacifier use

Prolonged pacifier or bottle use can also affect the palate and tooth positioning. Pacifiers are generally preferred to digit sucking for infant self-soothing; they decrease the risk of Sudden Infant Death Syndrome (SIDS) and are easier to discontinue in toddlers. Anticipatory guidance includes transition to cup use at age 12 months and limiting the pacifier to brief times when soothing is needed such as naps or bedtime. Older studies noted a strong correlation between prolonged bottle feeding and pacifier use with malocclusion and other bite abnormalities.[12] However, more recent meta-analyses have shown a less-decisive correlation and the presence of confounding bias.[13,14] Thus, the American Academy of Pediatric Dentistry now holds a more lenient stance on pacifiers in particular, but notes that prolonged pacifier use can lead to a need for intervention like a mouth appliance.[15]

Mouth breathing

Mouth breathing can result from functional or anatomic blockage in the nasopharynx such as tonsil or adenoid hypertrophy, sinusitis, foreign bodies, septal deviation, or choanal atresia. If persistent, mouth breathing can lead to an open bite or malocclusion. A common yet treatable cause is allergic or irritant rhinitis. Refer the patient to ENT for evaluation if mouth breathing is not improved with intranasal corticosteroid and/or oral antihistamines.[16]

Hyperdontia

Hyperdontia, or supernumerary teeth, can occur unilaterally or bilaterally. The most common presentation involves the permanent dentition in maxillary position. Another common location is between the central incisors, as a single extra tooth referred to as mesiodens. In primary dentition, the lateral incisors are the most common location with an incidence of 1% in typically developing children and 40% to 70% in children with orofacial clefts.[16]

Acquired Conditions: Infections

Caries

Dental caries are the most common chronic infection of childhood. In the United States, 24% of children aged 2 to 4 years have had caries, with the prevalence rising to 56% of children at the age of 15 years. Caries can have a significant negative impact on the quality of life, leading to pain, secondary infections, missed school days, and undesirable cosmesis. Furthermore, children from poor and/or minority families are more likely to suffer from caries and their complications.[17] The primary care provider is likely to frequently encounter caries and can serve roles in both prevention and management of this condition.

Pathogenesis of caries

The oral cavity experiences a range of dynamic conditions. Homeostasis of the oral cavity relies on a balance of factors, the imbalances of which can predispose to the development of caries. A useful conceptual model known as the caries balance explores these factors, with an equilibrium maintained between protective and pathologic factors. Protective factors include salivary flow and components, fluoride and other restorative ions, and antibacterial agents. Pathologic factors include acid-producing oral flora, the frequency and duration of exposure to fermentable carbohydrates, and altered salivary composition or flow.[18,19]

Mineralization equilibrium: The carbonated hydroxyapatite of enamel and dentin can be eroded by changing conditions in the oral cavity, leading to demineralization. Acidic environments enhance this demineralization, as carbonate inclusions in the crystal structure make tooth material vulnerable to acid erosion. Under appropriate conditions of pH and available calcium and phosphate, saliva can subsequently remineralize the crystal lattice of hydroxyapatite before the formation of a tooth cavity. The additional presence of fluoride ions can replace carbonate ions in the crystal structure during remineralization, creating a much more acid-resistant material. Conversely, nutrient deficiencies leading to hypomineralization, or congenital abnormalities such as enamel hypoplasia, can contribute to cariogenic demineralization.[18]

Fermentable carbohydrates: The presence of carbohydrates in the oral cavity contributes to the creation of an acidic environment via fermentation by-products of oral flora. The oral flora can metabolize numerous carbohydrates; glucose, sucrose, and fructose are commonly implicated cariogenic carbohydrates. Sucrose, specifically, can be problematic. Oral microbes can polymerize sucrose into a sticky polysaccharide, glucan, which persists in the oral cavity.[20] Glucan both increases the adhesion of cariogenic bacteria to the tooth surface and provides a long-lasting source of fermentable substrate, which is metabolized into acidic by-products, long after feeding has ceased.

The duration of exposure to carbohydrates, rather than the absolute quantity of carbohydrates consumed, correlates strongly with the risk of caries. During feeding, the oral pH drops quickly and typically takes between 30 and 90 minutes to return to preprandial levels. Sticky or long-lasting candies and bottles of sugary beverages retained through naps or sleep all have a greater cariogenic potential than other foods consumed in shorter periods.[18]

The presence of cariogenic bacteria, capable of fermenting carbohydrates into organic acids, is also critical to caries formation. Mutans group streptococci (*Streptococcus mutans, Streptococcus sobrinus,* and so forth) typically initiate the process. These acid-tolerant bacteria are prodigious acid fermenters, capable of clinging to dental enamel. Subsequent colonization by lactobacilli leads to further acid production and demineralization, and eventual invasion of the dentin and cavity formation.[2,18] It is worthwhile to note that vertical transmission does seem to occur in mutans group streptococci, leading to increased risk in offspring of adults with a history of caries.[21]

Salivary flow and composition: Saliva has multiple carioprotective characteristics. The mechanical flow of saliva dissolves carbohydrates and can wash bacteria off the teeth. The presence of dissolved ions can facilitate remineralization. Antibacterial compounds and immunoglobulins interfere with oral flora propagation and adhesion. Salivary proteins and lipids contribute to the formation of a protective pellicle on dental surfaces, reducing exposure to acid and also reducing bacterial adhesion.[22] Saliva also offers a buffering capacity against pH changes. Although an uncommon cause of caries when considered alone, alterations in salivary function can be cariogenic. Medications or diseases that cause xerostomia can predispose a patient to caries formation.

Early childhood caries

Early childhood caries (ECC), also known as bottle caries, is an early and aggressive form of tooth decay precipitated by inappropriate bottle-feeding habits. Infants and toddlers given carbohydrate-rich beverages such as Kool-Aid or sodas in a bottle, or inappropriately sugar-rich solids, can develop substantial caries; this can especially be driven by prolonged exposures such as all-day sippers or allowing a child to fall asleep with their bottle. Severity varies by the age, the number of teeth affected, and the tooth surface involved. Involvement of any smooth tooth surface is considered severe.[23] Even when treated, ECC is associated with a higher risk of more extensive adult caries. Education, thorough examination, and early establishment of a dental home both play important roles in reducing this condition.

Pulpitis

Caries in their most basic manifestation are typically asymptomatic; however, progression of cavitary disease eventually leads to the destruction of a bulk of the tooth and invasion of the dental pulp; this leads to inflammation and can cause substantial pain. Further extension of the infection can involve the alveolar space and alveolar bone, leading to dental abscess formation.

Dental abscess

Whether by extension of caries and pulpitis, translocated oral flora secondary to trauma, as sequalae of periodontal disease, or progression of failed restorative dentistry, abscess formation can occur. Either periodontal or periapical abscess formation is possible, presenting with pain, swelling, and sometimes fever. These infections are typically polymicrobial, with both aerobic and anaerobic flora involved. Common species include viridans group streptococci, *Fusobacterium,* and *Prevotella.*[24] Lacking prompt intervention, extension of dental abscesses can lead to a variety of deep tissue infections, sepsis, and other conditions beyond the scope of this article. Even barring such complications, however, painful dental abscesses can have a significant impact on quality of life, communication, and nutrition.

Treatment

Management of caries is best accomplished with an experienced dentist. Given the poor compliance of younger children, a pediatric dentist or a general dentist with significant pediatric care experience may be indicated, and sedation may be required. Restoration with amalgam, composites, or a crown can all ameliorate tooth damage after the infected tissue has been removed. Dental pain can often be relieved using nonsteroidal anti-inflammatory drugs, although opioid pain control may be required for severe cases. Although bacteria play a large role in cariogenesis, prophylactic use of antimicrobials is of limited value; chlorhexidine gluconate mouthwash can be used to suppress mutans group bacteria, but recolonization typically occurs within 2 weeks of treatment completion. As such, chlorhexidine typically serves a short- to medium-term adjunctive therapy for dental infections.

Dental abscesses also require definitive dental management, often with a root canal or dental extraction; however, this is accomplished after treatment of the infection, by surgical drainage and debridement and/or antibiotic therapy. Some cases of pulpitis may have sufficient bacterial involvement to require antibiotic treatment in addition to analgesics to achieve adequate pain control. Typical indications for antibiotics include fever, lymphadenopathy, or evidence of soft tissue involvement such as facial swelling. Oral penicillin is the typical drug of choice. Amoxicillin can be used for younger children when palatability is a concern. For those with penicillin allergies, clindamycin may be used, or cephalosporins can be considered given the low risk for cross-reactivity. Severe or extensive infections can be managed with extended β-lactam-resistant antibiotics such as amoxicillin-clavulanic acid.

Acquired Conditions: Dental Trauma

Dental trauma is common in childhood, with approximately 10% of children aged 18 months to 18 years experiencing some form of dental trauma. A variety of circumstances contribute, with falls and child abuse common in toddlerhood, accidents in school-aged children, and fights, sport injuries, and motor vehicle accidents predominant in adolescence. Anatomic variants such as prominent front teeth or craniofacial anomalies or neuromuscular or developmental abnormalities (eg, hypotonia) increase the risk of dental trauma in childhood. Maxillary incisors are the most commonly damaged teeth.[2] Injuries to periodontal structures, the maxilla, or the mandible can occur with or without tooth damage and must be considered, but many of these injuries are uncommon and will not be addressed here.

Regardless of the type of tooth injury, it is helpful to identify whether the affected teeth are from the primary or permanent dentition.[25]

Fractures

Tooth fractures are a common occurrence and can be divided into 2 general categories. Uncomplicated fractures only involve the hard structures of the tooth; complicated fractures extend into the dental pulp space. Such fractures expose the pulp to bacterial contamination, leading to an increased risk of both pulpitis and poor overall outcomes.

Both obvious and suspected occult tooth fractures require prompt evaluation by a dentist for a thorough clinical examination, potentially assisted with radiographs. Superficial damage to the enamel (crazing) is possible without obvious altered tooth structure. This condition can be difficult to identify without a formal dental examination and requires periodic reevaluation because of the increased risk of caries. With true fractures, recovery of the damaged tooth fragment or fragments if possible followed by a gentle rinsing and transportation in an isotonic solution can be helpful in restoration.

Displacements

Teeth are also often displaced by trauma; these displacements can be categorized as follows. Subluxation injuries leave the tooth in its normal anatomic position but loosened within the alveolar space. Extrusion injuries typically leave the tooth displaced lingually, with an associated alveolar wall fracture. Intrusion injuries drive the tooth deeper into the alveolar socket, sometimes leading to the false impression of a missing tooth that can only be located on radiographs. Finally, avulsion injuries, also known as a "knocked-out" tooth, completely displace the tooth from the alveolar socket.[26]

Management of subluxation, intrusion, and extrusion injuries are similar in that repositioning and/or stabilization of the tooth in the alveolar socket is required to facilitate healing. All these injuries carry a risk of pulp injury and subsequent necrosis; however, intrusions and extrusions have a substantially higher risk of complication and the need for endodontic treatment. Furthermore, extruded primary teeth are often extracted because of a high risk of subsequent interference with permanent dentition.[2]

Avulsed teeth are a time-sensitive issue. Avulsed primary teeth should not be reimplanted before the dental evaluation, whereas avulsed permanent teeth fare far better with prompt reimplantation.[25] Teeth replanted within 20 minutes have a good recovery rate, whereas those replanted more than 2 hours later have a high complication and failure rate.[2] The displaced tooth should be recovered promptly if possible, rinsed, and gently placed back in the socket, although it may still appear slightly extruded. If replanting is not possible, storage in a cold isotonic solution such as milk or normal saline will be helpful. Regardless, immediate dental evaluation is warranted as stabilization and endodontic treatment will be required for satisfactory outcomes.

Prevention

Many forms of dental trauma are avoidable, and the risks of some injuries can be modified. Mouth guards should be recommended for contact sports. Helmets should be recommended for wheeled activities such as biking; helmets with face guards can be used for children at high risk or for high-risk sports or sporting positions (eg, hockey goalies, baseball catchers). Furthermore, general good dental hygiene practices can keep teeth strong and more resilient to trauma.

Dental Best Practices and Preventative Care

As with most aspects of good health, prevention is the best approach to dental disease. The American Academy of Pediatrics (AAP) Section on Oral Health and the American Dental Association have recommendations, policy statements, and toolkits available for primary care providers available free online; these are a great resource for primary care providers seeking to implement oral health screening and treatment into their practice. Among the most important of these recommendations is that clinicians should perform a dental risk assessment and apply fluoride, starting at 6 months of age.

Dental risk assessment

The AAP recommends performing a dental risk assessment at the 6- and 9-month well child visits, where counseling and anticipatory guidance can be given regarding feeding habits, hygiene, fluoride, and establishing a dental home. The dental risk assessment should also be performed for any child without a dental home identified at the 12- through 30-month, 3-year, and 6-year visits. Risk factors and protective factors are identified in the dental risk assessment. There is a free tool available from the AAP to facilitate screening.

Risk factors include continual bottle/sippy cup use; access to beverages other than water between meals; frequent snacking with sugar or refined carbohydrates; special health care needs; and poor maternal oral health, for example, caries within the past 12 months; or lack of a dental home. Clinical risk factors include assessment for active dental caries, calcification, visible plaque, restorative fillings, or gingivitis present on examination.

Protective factors include brushing teeth twice daily with age-appropriate amounts of fluoridated toothpaste, a dental home established by age 12 months with regular visits every 6 months, topical fluoride applied every 6 months, and a fluoridated water source or fluoride supplement. Healthy-appearing teeth free of the above risk factors on examination should be noted.

Creating a plan based on the dental risk assessment is essential, and counseling should be provided to the caregiver—and child, if age appropriate. For caregivers with active dental caries, encourage the caregiver to seek care, and to avoid sharing utensils, cups, or similar objects to prevent transmission of odontogenic bacteria.[27]

The primary care provider should also provide counseling at all preventative health visits to encourage good oral health habits.

Good dental hygiene

The American Academy of Pediatric Dentistry recommends cleaning an infant's teeth with a small-head soft-bristled brush and a rice grain-sized smear of fluoride-containing toothpaste twice daily. Children aged 3 years and older with the ability to spit may use a pea-sized amount of fluoride-containing toothpaste twice daily[15] (**Figs. 2** and **3**).

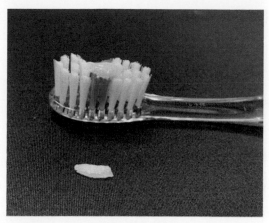

Fig. 2. Appropriate quantity of toothpaste for infants.

Healthy dietary habits

Families may not realize that good dietary practices impact dental health as well as nutritional health. Encourage 3 meals per day and 2 to 3 discrete snacks per day from 9 to 12 months of age onward, with plenty of fresh vegetables offered. Continual snacking of carbohydrate-based foods in particular worsens the risk of cariogenesis. In the same way, it is important to limit high-sugar foods and sweetened beverages. Offer cow's milk only with meals and water between meals. As much as possible, avoid cow's milk before bed or in the middle of the night; if it is given at these times, brush the teeth after.[28]

Increase fluoride exposure

Several studies have shown a strong correlation between fluoride exposure, particularly in drinking water, and protection from dental caries.[10] In areas where it is available, drink fluoridated tap water; less than 6 months of age, use it to mix formula,

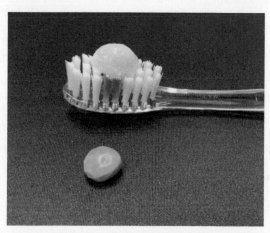

Fig. 3. Appropriate quantity of toothpaste for children aged 3 years and older.

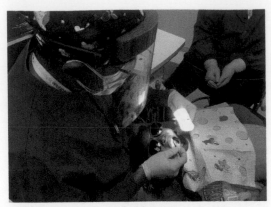

Fig. 4. Appropriate positioning for dental fluoride application.

and once older than 6 months of age, drink water as appropriate. Once the teeth have erupted, clean the teeth twice daily with appropriate quantities of fluoride-containing toothpaste. Primary care offices can also support good dental hygiene by having office toothbrush giveaways and by providing fluoride treatments.

In-office fluoride application with 5% sodium fluoride every 3 to 6 months, depending on risk factors, is recommended by the US Preventative Services Task Force. This application is covered by most insurance and is a quick and effective way to reduce the incidence of dental caries by up to 35%.[10] Best application is achieved from an above-the-head approach (**Fig. 4**), as in a dental office. For an infant or toddler, this positioning can be achieved with the child facing the caregiver with legs around the waist, laying back with the child's head on the caregiver's knees, and then the provider sitting knee-to-knee with the caregiver. The caregiver can then assist by holding the child's hands. Dry the teeth with gauze or tissue, and gently brush the fluoride on all dental surfaces. Counsel to avoid food or drink for 30 minutes, and then only consume soft, nonabrasive foods for the remainder of the day.

Regular dental care and the placement of sealants

Encourage patients to establish a dental home by 12 months of age and maintain regular dental visits every 6 months. The American Academy of Pediatric Dentistry published a 2016 guideline[29] recommending the use of pit and fissure sealants on the primary and permanent molars of children and adolescents. A 2016 systematic review[30] showed that sealants were more effective at caries prevention than topical fluoride varnish alone.

Additional pediatric-specific oral health pearls

- Encourage the treatment of the caregiver's dental caries to prevent transmission of cariogenic bacteria to infants.[21]
- Discourage bottle use past 12 months of age and begin counseling on pacifier cessation at 12 months.
- Encourage the use of mouth guards for contact sports.[31]

SUMMARY AND KEY CLINICAL CARE POINTS

Oral health is an important part of the preventative medicine encounter, and clinicians should be prepared to monitor normal dental development, screen for abnormalities, and understand the basic care of dental infections and trauma. In addition, the clinician should be mindful that dental caries are the most common chronic disease of childhood, and as such, every preventative visit should involve a dental risk assessment and counseling on dental hygiene practices.

CLINICS CARE POINTS

---

1. Perform a dental risk assessment at routine well child visits.
2. Use the preventative visit to provide counseling to encourage healthy preventive habits.
   a. Drink fluoridated tap water.
   b. Clean erupted teeth twice daily with appropriate quantities of fluoride-containing toothpaste: rice grain sized for infants and pea sized for children aged %3 years and older who can effectively spit.
   c. Encourage families to establish a dental home by age 1 year and recommend dental visits every 6 months.
   d. Limit sugar-sweetened beverages and carbohydrate snacks.
3. Provide fluoride treatments at routine well child visits, and up to every 3 months for children at high risk of caries.

ACKNOWLEDGMENTS

Thank you to Dr Nicole Bichir for providing **Figs. 1–4.**

REFERENCES

1. Martin B. Oral disorders. In: Zitelli BJ, McIntire SC, Nowalk AJ, editors. Zitelli and Davis' atlas of pediatric physical diagnosis. 6th edition. Philadelphia, PA: Elsevier; 2018. p. 775–802.
2. Tinanoff N. The oral cavity. In: Kliegman R, Lye PS, Bordini BJ, et al, editors. Nelson pediatric symptom-based diagnosis. Philadelphia, PA: Elsevier; 2018. p. 1529–38.
3. Michael LM, Marion P, Jonathan J, et al. Symptoms Associated With Infant Teething: A Prospective Study. Pediatrics 2000;105(4, Part 1 of 2):747–52.
4. Healthychildren.org. Baby Teething Pain. 2018. Available at: https://www.healthychildren.org/English/ages-stages/baby/teething-tooth-care/Pages/Teething-Pain.aspx. Accessed October 21, 2020.
5. Jaskoll T, Abichaker G, Jangaard N, et al. Cytomegalovirus inhibition of embryonic mouse tooth development: A model of the human amelogenesis imperfecta phenocopy. Arch Oral Biol 2008;53:405–15.
6. Ruchi A, Anand LS, Gagan T, et al. Dental manifestations of congenital rubella syndrome. BMJ Case Rep 2015;2015. bcr2015209382.
7. Nissanka-Jayasuriya EH, Odell EW, Phillips C. Dental Stigmata of Congenital Syphilis: A Historic Review With Present Day Relevance. Head Neck Pathol 2016;10(3):327–31.
8. Pernille EJ, Tine BH, Dorte H, et al. Prenatal exposure to antiepileptic drugs and dental agenesis. PLoS One 2014;9(1):e84420.
9. Guveli BT, Rosti RO, Guzeltas A, et al. Teratogenicity of antiepileptic drugs. Curr Opin Neurol 2017;15:19–27.
10. Brecher EA, Lewis CW. Infant Oral Health. Pediatr Clin North Am 2018;65(5):909–21.

11. Hampl M, Cela P, Szabo-Rogers HL, et al. Role of Primary Cilia in Odontogenesis. J dental Res 2017;96(9):965–74.

12. Hovorakova M, Lesot H, Peterka M, et al. Early development of the human dentition revisited. J Anat 2018;233:135–45.

13. Hermont AP, Martins CC, Zina LG, et al. Breastfeeding, bottle feeding practices and malocclusion in the primary dentition: a systematic review of cohort studies. Int J Environ Res Public Health 2015;12(3):3133–51.

14. Karin Michèle S, Remo K, Prasad N, et al. The effect of pacifier sucking on orofacial structures: a systematic literature review. Prog Orthod 2018;19(1):1–11.

15. Dentistry AAoP. Frequently Asked Questions (FAQ). Available at: https://www.aapd.org/resources/parent/faq/. Accessed October 29, 2020.

16. Jing Z, Mingmei M, Clarice SL, et al. Common dental diseases in children and malocclusion. Int J Oral Sci 2018;10(1):1–7.

17. Bruce AD, Gina T-E. Trends in Oral Health by Poverty Status as Measured by Healthy People 2010 Objectives. Public Health Rep 2010;125(6):817–30.

18. Featherstone JDB. The caries balance: the basis for caries management by risk assessment. Oral Health Prev Dent 2004;2(Suppl 1):259–64.

19. Featherstone JDB. The Caries Balance. Dimensions of Dental Hygiene. 2004. 2004. Available at: https://dimensionsofdentalhygiene.com/article/the-caries-balance/. Accessed October 24, 2020.

20. Kliegman R, Lye PS, Bordini BJ, et al. Nelson pediatric symptom-based diagnosis. Philadelphia, PA: Elsevier; 2018.

21. Douglass JM, Li Y, Tinanoff N. Association of Mutans Streptococci Between Caregivers and Their Children. Pediatr Dent 2008;30:375–87.

22. Siqueira WL, Custodio W, McDonald EE. New insights into the composition and functions of the acquired enamel pellicle. J Dent Res 2012;91:1110–8.

23. Ng MW. Chase II. Dental caries. In: Kline MW, editor. Rudolph's pediatrics. 23rd edition. New York: McGraw-Hill Education; 2018. p. 1647–50.

24. Shweta, Prakash SK. Dental abscess: A microbiological review. Dental Res J 2013;10(5):585–91.

25. Martof A, Martof A. Consultation with the specialist: dental care. Pediatr Rev 2001;22(1):13.

26. Keels MA, Section Oral H. Management of dental trauma in a primary care setting. Pediatrics 2014;133:E466–76.

27. Pediatrics AAo. Oral Health Risk Assessment Tool. 2011. Available at: https://www.aap.org/en-us/Documents/oralhealth_RiskAssessmentTool.pdf. Accessed October 25, 2020.

28. van Loveren C. Sugar Restriction for Caries Prevention: Amount and Frequency. Which Is More Important? Caries Res 2019;53(2):168–75.

29. Wright JT, Crall JJ, Fontana M, et al. Evidence-based clinical practice guideline for the use of pit-and-fissure sealants: A report of the American Dental Association and the American Academy of Pediatric Dentistry. J Am Dental Assoc 2016; 147(8):672–82.

30. Wright JT, Tampi MP, Graham L, et al. Sealants for preventing and arresting pit-and-fissure occlusal caries in primary and permanent molars: A systematic review of randomized controlled trials—a report of the American Dental Association and the American Academy of Pediatric Dentistry. J Am Dental Assoc 2016; 147(8):631–45.

31. Labella CR, Smith BW, Sigurdsson A. Effect of mouthguards on dental injuries and concussions in college basketball. Med Sci Sports Exerc 2002;34(1):41–4.

Common Pediatric Gastrointestinal Disorders

Jordan Hilgefort, MD, CAQSM[a,b,]*, Jonathan Newsom, MD, CAQSM[a,b]

KEYWORDS

- Gastrointestinal • Pediatric • Motility • Functional • Peristalsis

KEY POINTS

- Infectious diarrhea is most commonly viral in etiology, and treatment consists of supportive management.
- Diarrhea with antecedent use of antibiotics should raise concern for *Clostridioides difficile*.
- Diagnosis of ulcerative colitis imparts a markedly increased risk of colon cancer compared with a mildly increased risk with Crohn disease.
- Gastroesophageal reflux is very common in infancy and often resolves by age 6 to 12 months.
- Functional gastrointestinal disorders lack identifiable structural defects, and therefore do not require imaging studies for diagnosis.

INTRODUCTION

This article reviews common gastrointestinal (GI) disorders encountered in the outpatient pediatric setting with a focus on treatment and management directed by the clinician. Although this list of conditions is not comprehensive, it does serve to provide an extensive purview of various GI complaints and illnesses that the provider can expect to manage while caring for a pediatric population. We have chosen to concentrate our discussion by organizing each disorder into 1 of 3 general categories: infectious, inflammatory, and immunologic pathology; motility disorders; and functional GI disorders.

INFECTIOUS, INFLAMMATORY, AND IMMUNOLOGIC PATHOLOGY
Infection

Diarrhea
Although the most common cause of diarrhea in children is viral gastroenteritis, bacterial and parasitic infections may also be a trigger in this patient population.[1] Details

---

The authors have no commercial or financial conflicts of interest to disclose.
[a] Department of Family and Geriatric Medicine, University of Louisville, Louisville, KY, USA;
[b] Centers for Primary Care, 215 Central Avenue Suite 205, Louisville, KY 40208, USA
* Corresponding author.
E-mail address: jordan.hilgefort@louisville.edu

Prim Care Clin Office Pract 48 (2021) 443–459
https://doi.org/10.1016/j.pop.2021.04.008
0095-4543/21/© 2021 Elsevier Inc. All rights reserved.

surrounding onset, season of the year, and the course of illness may provide insight as to the offending agent. Treatment is generally supportive; however, in persistent cases, stool culture and antigen testing, as well as antibiotics, may be required. It is important to remember that nonenteric infections can also stimulate diarrhea, the likes of which include urinary tract infections, acute otitis media, and pneumonia (**Table 1**).

Colitis
Clostridioides difficile colitis occurs due to overgrowth of this bacterium and accumulation of bacterial toxins in the bowel.

Symptoms:

- Watery diarrhea
- Abdominal pain
- Fever
- Chance of progress to toxic megacolon or shock

Risk factors:

- Antecedent use of antibiotics
- Acid suppression (eg, proton pump inhibitors)
- Malignancy
- Inflammatory bowel disease
- Cystic fibrosis
- Immunodeficiency
- Enteric feeding tubes[2]

Stool culture, stool antigen, toxin testing, or polymerase chain reaction are used for diagnosis but should be exploited in cases when considerable clinical suspicion exists in the setting of copious diarrhea.[2] Initial treatment includes oral antibiotics (vancomycin, fidaxomicin, or metronidazole) but may become more complex with persistence of infection.

Necrotizing enterocolitis
Necrotizing enterocolitis (NEC) is ischemic necrosis of the bowel mucosa that progresses to severe inflammation, bacterial overgrowth, and the presence of gas in

Table 1
Common sources, symptoms, and risk factors for diarrhea

Etiology	Common Organisms	Symptoms	Risk Factors
Viral	*Rotavirus* *Norovirus* Adenovirus	Nonbloody diarrhea Vomiting Fever	Contaminated food or water
Bacterial	*Escherichia coli* *Salmonella* *Shigella* *C difficile* *Campylobacter jejuni* *Yersinia enterocolitica*	Bloody diarrhea Mucus in stools Tenesmus Fever Severe abdominal pain	Farm animal exposure Contaminated meat
Parasitic	*Giardia* *Cryptosporidium* Amebiasis	Nonbloody diarrhea Abdominal cramping	Immune suppression Immigration Recent travel Camping Processed meats Meats from farm animals

the bowel wall or portal circulation. NEC is a common emergency in newborn infants, and the incidence is inversely proportional to the gestational age at birth.[3]

Features of presentation:

- Sudden decrease in feeding
- Abdominal distension
- Abdominal tenderness
- Bilious vomiting
- Diarrhea
- Hematochezia

Laboratory studies may exhibit anemia and thrombocytopenia. Radiographic evidence of NEC includes abnormal gas patterns and dilated bowel loops, as well as pneumatosis intestinalis. Rarely, pneumoperitoneum may occur with bowel rupture. Workup includes a complete blood cell count, coagulation studies, and metabolic panels. The Modified Bell Staging Criteria for NEC in neonates is available to aid in diagnosis and incorporates systemic, abdominal, and radiographic signs for staging.[3] Treatment is supportive for Bell stages I and II and involves use of antibiotics, total parenteral nutrition, gastric decompression, bowel rest, and serial examinations. More severe disease is treated surgically. Despite advances in treatment, the mortality rate for infants with Bell stage II or III NEC is 23.5%.[3,4]

Inflammatory Disorders

Inflammatory Bowel Disease

Inflammatory bowel disease (IBD) is divided into Crohn disease (Crohn) and ulcerative colitis (UC). Crohn can involve any portion of the GI tract from the oral cavity to the anus, although the most common areas affected are the ileum and cecum.[6] A hallmark of the disease is transmural inflammation. Conversely, UC is characterized by inflammation of the mucosal layer and progresses in a continuous, retrograde manner from rectum to colon.[6]

Diagnosis should be obtained through colonoscopy with random biopsies. Imaging of the upper GI tract can be useful in aiding the differentiation between UC and Crohn, and this can be accomplished via magnetic resonance imaging, computed tomography, or upper GI with small bowel follow-through imaging. Complications from IBD can include fistula, peritonitis, abscess formation, and small bowel obstruction. Treatment is multifactorial and can include aminosalicylates, antibiotics, corticosteroids, and immunomodulators. Nutritional supplementation may be required as well (**Table 2**).[5–7]

Immunologic Disorders

Celiac disease (gluten-sensitive enteropathy)

Celiac disease is an autoimmune disorder stimulated by exposure to dietary gluten, present in wheat, rye, and barley grains. Exposure to gluten provokes chronic inflammation in the small bowel, inducing atrophy of intestinal villi and ultimately leading to malabsorption (**Table 3**).

Cow's milk protein intolerance

This condition involves hypersensitivity to cow's milk protein, present in 5% to 15% of infants.[8] The sensitivity can be immunoglobulin E (IgE) or non-IgE mediated. IgE-mediated sensitivity carries an increased risk for development of extraintestinal atopic conditions such as asthma and eczema. Mild symptoms range from vomiting, regurgitation, diarrhea, and hematochezia, to name a few. However, severe symptoms can entail the likes of failure to thrive, angioedema, or anaphylaxis. Diagnosis is largely

Table 2
Crohn disease versus ulcerative colitis

Feature	Crohn Disease	Ulcerative Colitis
Site	Terminal ileum Can occur anywhere from mouth to anus	Rectum
Progression	Irregular	Proximally
Inflammation	Transmural	Mucosal
Symptoms	Abdominal cramping	Bloody diarrhea
Complications	Fistulas Abscesses Obstructions Extraintestinal manifestations	Hemorrhage Toxic megacolon

Radiographic findings	String sign on barium
	    radiography
		Lead pipe colon on
		    barium radiography

Colon cancer risk	Mild increase	Marked increase

Data from Refs.[5–7]

clinical and should carry a high index of suspicion. Recognition of symptoms following ingestion of cow's milk is key, although formal allergy testing and identification of IgE for cow's milk protein may play a role. A trial of elimination of cow's milk from maternal diet (if breastfeeding) or formula is the mainstay of management. Reintroduction of cow's milk should be attempted after 4 weeks and if symptoms have resolved, may continue in perpetuity.[8]

MOTILITY DISORDERS
Disorders of Peristalsis

Hirschsprung disease
Also known as congenital aganglionic bowel disease, Hirschsprung disease (HD) causes unopposed contraction of the distal colon, resulting in obstruction of fecal contents and proximal colonic dilation; it is caused by an embryologic failure of

Table 3
Clinical features of celiac disease

Clinical features	• Rash: dermatitis herpetiformis • Diarrhea • Weight loss • Low bone mineral density • Iron deficiency • Neuropathy
Diagnosis	• Anti–tissue transglutaminase antibodies • Confirmation with small bowel biopsy
Treatment	• Gluten-free diet • Corticosteroids • Immunomodulators

Data from Pelkowski, TD, Veira AJ. Celiac disease: diagnosis and management. Amer Fam Phys. 2014:89(2); 99-105.

ganglionic progenitor cells originating from the neural crest to appropriately migrate to the distal colon.

Epidemiology:

- The most common organic cause of constipation in otherwise healthy children
- However, HD represents less than 5% of cases of childhood constipation[9,10]
- Approximately 1 in 5000 live births[9]
- Affects males 3 to 5 times more commonly than females
- Associated with a family history of the disorder in 80% of the cases

Clinical features:

- Failure to pass meconium stool within 48 hours of birth (depending on the severity of condition)
- Chronic constipation
- Bilious emesis
- Abdominal distension
- Failure to thrive

Early recognition is key, and although rectal biopsy is the gold standard of diagnosis, barium enema often precedes biopsy. Surgical resection of the aganglionic portion of bowel represents definitive treatment.

Infantile hypertrophic pyloric stenosis

Infantile hypertrophic pyloric stenosis involves congenital hypertrophy and hypertonicity of the pylorus muscle causing gastric outlet obstruction and resultant projectile vomiting in infants.

Epidemiology:

- Approximately 1 per 250 live births[9]
- Affects males 4 to 6 times more commonly than females
- An estimated 1.5-fold increased risk in first-born children[11]
- Increased risk imparted by exposure to erythromycin and azithromycin, particularly within the first 2 weeks of infancy[11]

Clinical features:

- Postprandial, nonbilious, projectile vomiting
- Development of symptoms between the ages of 3 and 6 weeks
- Irritable but hungry
- Dehydration
- Palpable mass superior and to the right of the umbilicus (olivelike mass)

Diagnosis may be suspected by laboratory perturbations, specifically hypochloremic, hypokalemic metabolic alkalosis. Abdominal ultrasonography is the study of choice, although barium upper GI study may illustrate a narrow pyloric channel (string sign) indicating this disorder. Transection of the pylorus muscle fibers via partial pyloromyotomy is the treatment of this condition.

Malrotation and midgut volvulus

Malrotation and midgut volvulus is an anatomic abnormality in which the midgut twists around the superior mesenteric vasculature resulting in considerable potential for bowel obstruction and/or infarction. Malrotation occurs when the normal bowel rotation and fixation to the abdominal wall is interrupted during embryologic development. This failure of fixation and proper positioning of the bowels creates an environment wherein the bowel can freely twist on its central axis, leading to obstruction of the bowel lumen and vasculature.

Epidemiology:

- Approximately 1 in 500 live births
- Affects males twice as commonly as females[9]

Clinical features

- Sudden-onset abdominal pain
- Abdominal distension
- Bilious vomiting
- Blood-tinged stools

As symptoms can be nonspecific, initial workup generally begins with an abdominal radiograph, which may demonstrate proximal intestinal distension and obstruction with minimal to absent bowel gas. Nonetheless, upper GI series with oral contrast is the gold standard for diagnosis and should follow radiography when pathologic condition is suspected. Treatment is surgical—abdominal exploration, unraveling the gut, resection of nonviable segments of the intestines, and fixation of the gut to the abdominal wall to prevent recurrence.

Atresias

Atresia is congenital obstruction of the alimentary tract caused by an embryologic failure of the lumen to recanalize or a mesenteric vascular insult during gestation.

Epidemiology:

- Intestinal atresia is the most common cause of neonatal bowel obstruction
- Approximately 25% of cases are associated with Down syndrome[9]

Clinical features:

- Scaphoid abdomen with epigastric distension
- Vomiting
- Feeding intolerance
- Weight loss
- Failure to thrive

Abdominal radiograph illustrates air fluid levels, and in the case of duodenal atresia, in a classic pattern described as the double bubble sign. An intestinal contrast study pinpoints the region of atresia or stenosis. Nasogastric suctioning for abdominal decompression is used for initial management, whereas surgical resection and anastomosis of the affected segment of bowel is the conclusive treatment.

Intussusception

Intussusception is the invagination of a segment of intestine into a more distal portion of the intestine in a telescoping manner. A lead point is generally believed to stimulate the development of this pathologic condition. Common examples of lead points include Meckel diverticulum, a polyp, and lymphoma among others.

Epidemiology:

- Occurs in1 to 4 children per 1000
- Peak incidence between ages 5 and 9 months[9]
- The most common cause of bowel obstruction occurring after the neonatal period in children younger than 2 years[9]
- Ileocolic intussusception is the most common

Clinical features:

- Sudden-onset abdominal pain
- Vomiting
- Lethargy
- Bloody stools (classically described as currant jelly stools)
- Sausage-shaped palpable mass may be apparent in the right upper quadrant

Abdominal radiography is likely to reveal dilated loops of bowel or pneumoperitoneum if complicated by intestinal perforation. Abdominal ultrasonography may unreliably depict the area of intussusception. Air or contrast enema is both diagnostic and therapeutic, with an estimated success rate of 80% to 90%.[9] Operative reduction is pursued when enema fails or when evidence of peritonitis or pneumoperitoneum exists.

Disorders of Retroperistalsis

Gastroesophageal reflux

Gastroesophageal reflux (GER) a condition in which gastric contents transfer in a retrograde manner from the stomach into the esophagus. At baseline, the lower esophageal sphincter remains in a contracted state and provides a protective barrier between the esophagus and the highly acidic environment of the stomach. Upon swallowing, the esophagus transports food from the oropharynx to the stomach via coordinated waves of peristaltic contraction, which signal the normally contracted lower esophageal sphincter to relax, thereby allowing a food or liquid bolus to pass through the sphincter and enter into the stomach. GER occurs when the lower esophageal sphincter experiences transient relaxation without peristalsis, thus permitting gastric contents to enter the esophagus. Likewise, delayed gastric emptying may create an environment whereby gastric contents increasingly accumulate, causing gastric distension and inducing inappropriate, transient relaxation of the lower esophageal sphincter. This dysfunction becomes pathologic when GI or pulmonary symptoms develop as a result of exposure to gastric contents, at which point this condition is referred to as gastroesophageal reflux disease (GERD).

Epidemiology:

- GER has an incidence of up to 60% in infancy
- Approximately 10% of infants with GER develop GERD[9]

Clinical features

- GER
  - Spitting up or vomiting, often described as happy spitters
- GERD
  - Emesis
  - Torticollis and arching of the back (Sandifer syndrome) caused by painful esophagitis
  - Feeding refusal
  - Failure to thrive
  - Constant hunger (milk may act as a buffer to limit acidic irritation)
  - Endorsement of midepigastric pain in older children
  - Nausea (particularly upon awakening)
  - Hoarseness
  - Halitosis
  - Cough and/or wheezing

Diagnosis largely entails clinical recognition of symptoms, although evaluation for GERD can include one or more of the following: barium GI study, scintigraphy, esophageal pH measurement, endoscopy, and bronchoscopy with alveolar lavage (to confirm aspiration). Although GER generally resolves without intervention by age 6 to 12 months, symptoms that persist beyond age 1 year and older children developing GERD are unlikely to experience spontaneous resolution. Management is multifactorial, encompassing the following measures:

Treatment:

- Upright positioning, sitting up, elevating the head of the bed
- Frequent, small meals
- Thicken feeds—infant cereal or commercial thickeners
- Acid inhibitors—antacids, H_2 blockers, proton pump inhibitors
- Metoclopramide—increase sphincter tone and promote gastric emptying
- Surgical intervention for recalcitrant cases
  - Nissen fundoplication
  - Gastric antroplasty

FUNCTIONAL GASTROINTESTINAL DISORDERS

Functional gastrointestinal disorders (FGID) are broadly considered GI ailments featuring a lack of structural disease to correlate with patient symptoms.[12–16] The Rome Foundation, responsible for establishing sets of diagnostic criteria for identifying the various disorders comprising FGID, characterizes these ailments as "disorders of gut-brain interaction." The predominant theory regarding FGID references the biopsychosocial model and contends that disturbances in mood, behavior, stress, social circumstance, thoughts, and emotional well-being, among others, stimulate an imbalance between the mind and body and result in pathologic condition.[17,18]

Functional Nausea and Vomiting Disorders

Nausea is innately a subjective sensation, whereas vomiting is a critical anatomic reflex in response to infectious, inflammatory, neoplastic, metabolic, or noxious stimuli believed to provide some degree of protection to the alimentary tract. These set of disorders represent dysfunction in regulation of nausea and vomiting, among others.

Cyclic vomiting syndrome

Cyclic vomiting syndrome (CVS) is a disorder impacting an estimated 1% of children with typical onset occurring between ages 3.5 to 7 years.[17,18] Although testing is not necessary to make the diagnosis, onset at an earlier age should prompt consideration of physical or metabolic abnormalities. A separate but similar disorder sharing features of CVS is cannabinoid hyperemesis syndrome (CHS), a condition whereby frequent use of cannabis stimulates abdominal pain, nausea, and recurrent episodes of emesis. Consideration of this condition should be exercised particularly in an adolescent patient population presenting with frequent nausea and vomiting. Notably, showering or bathing in hot water provides transient relief of symptoms in patients with CHS. Assessing the influence of hot water on regulation of symptoms is thereby useful in differentiating this condition from CVS. (**Table 4**).

Functional nausea and functional vomiting

Recently established as their own separate diagnostic entities, functional nausea and functional vomiting may occur in isolation or in tandem.[19] Distinction should

Table 4
Cyclic vomiting syndrome Rome IV diagnostic criteria and treatment considerations

Rome IV diagnostic criteria	All of the following must be present for diagnosis: 1. No fewer than 2 discrete periods of intense, persistent nausea highlighted by paroxysmal episodes of vomiting lasting for hours to days over a 6-mo time frame 2. Episodes are stereotypical for each patient 3. Episodes are separated by weeks to months with return to baseline health in the interim 4. Symptoms cannot be fully explained by another medical condition

Treatment recommendations	• Acute management consists of rehydration and pharmacologic treatment:
	  ○ Cyproheptadine for children <5 years old
	  ○ Amitriptyline for children >5 years old
	• Prophylactic management with propranolol
	• Adjunctive management: coenzyme Q10 & L-carnitine
	• Cognitive behavioral therapy
	• Acupuncture

Adapted from Hyams JS, Di Lorenzo C, Saps M, et al. Childhood functional gastrointestinal disorders: child/adolescent. *Gastroenterology.* 2016;150:1456–68; with permission.

be made between these disorders and functional dyspepsia (FD), of which the latter involves nausea and/or vomiting associated with concomitant abdominal pain (**Tables 5 and 6**).

There remains a lack of evidence-based treatment of both these disorders; however, cognitive behavioral therapy and hypnotherapy have been proposed. Cyproheptadine has successfully been used for the treatment of FD, and by extrapolation, may consequently also provide benefit for these conditions.

Rumination syndrome

Rumination syndrome is the repetitive regurgitation of gastric contents, which are rechewed and either swallowed or spit out, typically shortly after eating. Estimates of prevalence are difficult to assess given that parents are often unaware of the occurrence; however, adolescent girls are believed to be at higher risk. The process of rumination is most often volitional and in response to either physical discomfort or

Table 5
Functional nausea Rome IV diagnostic criteria and treatment considerations

Rome IV diagnostic criteria	Functional nausea requires all of the following for 2 mo: 1. Nausea occurring at least twice per week, and generally unrelated to consumption of meals 2. Not reliably associated with vomiting 3. Symptoms cannot be fully explained by another medical condition

Adapted from Hyams JS, Di Lorenzo C, Saps M, et al. Childhood functional gastrointestinal disorders: child/adolescent. *Gastroenterology.* 2016;150:1456–68; with permission.

Table 6	
Functional vomiting Rome IV diagnostic criteria and treatment considerations	
Rome IV diagnostic criteria	Functional vomiting requires all of the following: 1. One or more episodes of vomiting on average per week 2. Absence of evidence for self-induced vomiting, an eating disorder, or rumination syndrome 3. Symptoms cannot be fully explained by another medical condition

Adapted from Hyams JS, Di Lorenzo C, Saps M, et al. Childhood functional gastrointestinal disorders: child/adolescent. *Gastroenterology*. 2016;150:1456–1468; with permission.

behavioral impulse. Contraction of abdominal musculature provokes an increase in intragastric pressure and forces gastric contents through the lower esophageal sphincter upward to the mouth. Recent infection or traumatic psychological episode is often the triggers for onset of rumination (**Table 7**).

Aerophagia

Aerophagia is the excessive air swallowing that occurs in an estimated 4% of children.[19] Air progressively fills the intraluminal space of the stomach, often results in inordinate belching and flatulence, and can be a source of abdominal pain (**Table 8**).

Functional Abdominal Pain Disorders

Abdominal pain is one of the most common GI complaints in pediatric and adult patients alike; nonetheless, a definitive, physical defect responsible for the impending pathologic condition can be identified in a mere 1 in 10 pediatric patients.[16] These types of abdominal pain, lacking a distinct abnormality, are more precisely characterized as functional abdominal pain disorders (FAPD). The diagnosis of one of these conditions requires the absence of evidence for inflammatory, metabolic, infectious, or anatomic pathology, which would more appropriately account for the patient's abdominal pain.[17]

Table 7	
Rumination syndrome Rome IV diagnostic criteria and treatment considerations	

Rome IV diagnostic criteria	All of the following for at least 2 mo:
	1. Recurrent regurgitation, rechewing, and swallowing or expulsion of food that:
	  a. Begins shortly after consumption of a meal
	  b. Does not occur during sleep
	2. Not preceded by retching
	3. Symptoms cannot be fully explained by another medical condition

Treatment recommendations	Interdisciplinary behavioral interventions designed to alter learned habits: psychology, clinical nutrition, therapeutic recreation, massage therapy, and child life services are options used for treatment, often in an inpatient setting

Adapted from Hyams JS, Di Lorenzo C, Saps M, et al. Childhood functional gastrointestinal disorders: child/adolescent. *Gastroenterology*. 2016;150:1456–68; with permission.

Table 8	
Aerophagia Rome IV diagnostic criteria and treatment considerations	
Rome IV diagnostic criteria	All of the following for at least 2 mo before diagnosis: 1. Excessive air swallowing 2. Abdominal distension due to air swallowing throughout the day 3. Repetitive eructation and/or flatulence 4. Symptoms cannot be fully explained by another medical condition
Treatment recommendations	There are no evidence-based guidelines to direct treatment, but recommendations include behavioral therapies and psychotherapy, as well as consideration of benzodiazepines

Adapted from Hyams JS, Di Lorenzo C, Saps M, et al. Childhood functional gastrointestinal disorders: child/adolescent. *Gastroenterology.* 2016;150:1456–68; with permission.

Functional dyspepsia

FD represents one or more of a predictable set of upper abdominal symptoms believed to be associated with dysfunction in gastric motility, oversensitization of the gastric mucosa, inflammation, and/or genetic predisposition; nonetheless, the pathophysiology of this condition remains unclear because the spectrum of this disorder is rather heterogeneous. One study also found that FD developed as residuum of acute bacterial gastroenteritis in 24% of children previously infected, although a similar correlation was not established with viral gastroenteritis.[19] There are 2 predominant subtypes of FD: postprandial distress syndrome and epigastric pain syndrome (**Table 9**).

Table 9	
Functional dyspepsia Rome IV diagnostic criteria and treatment considerations	
Rome IV diagnostic criteria	One or more of the following at least 4 d per month, for a period of at least 2 mo before diagnosis: 1. Postprandial fullness 2. Early satiety 3. Epigastric pain or burning not associated with defecation 4. Symptoms cannot be fully explained by another medical condition
Treatment recommendations	No large, double-blind, placebo-controlled trials exist to support evidence-based treatment options; however, recommendations include: • Avoidance of caffeine, as well as spicy and fatty foods • Histamine H2 receptor antagonists and proton pump inhibitors • Cyproheptadine • For recalcitrant cases, consideration of low-dose tricyclic antidepressants (eg, amitriptyline, imipramine)

Adapted from Hyams JS, Di Lorenzo C, Saps M, et al. Childhood functional gastrointestinal disorders: child/adolescent. *Gastroenterology.* 2016;150:1456–68; with permission.

Irritable bowel syndrome

Irritable bowel syndrome (IBS) is characterized by abdominal pain associated with a change in bowel habits. With an estimated incidence of 10% to 15%, IBS represents the most common source of intermittent abdominal pain in children.[20] Prevailing hypotheses regarding pathophysiology of this condition draw strong correlation to psychosocial stressors, including anxiety, depression, and alterations in mood. Similar to FD, dysfunction in gastric motility, oversensitization of the gastric and intestinal mucosa, and inflammation are implicated in this condition. In addition, evidence of mutation in the gut microbiome has been recognized in patients with IBS, although it is uncertain whether this is a cause or an outcome of the condition (**Table 10**).

Abdominal migraine

Abdominal migraine (AM) entails intermittent, self-limited episodes of intense abdominal pain associated with migrainelike symptoms. Triggers (eg, stress, insomnia, fatigue), symptoms, and alleviating factors tend to be immutable. Studies suggest an incidence between 1% and 23% (**Table 11**).

Functional abdominal pain—not otherwise specified

Functional abdominal pain—not otherwise specified (FAP-NOS) provides a diagnosis for patients with abdominal pain who fail to meet the specified criteria for the aforementioned FAPD but are also devoid of an organic source of pathology or a specific physiologic process to account for symptoms. The syndrome associated with this type of pain, previously described as functional abdominal pain syndrome, has now more aptly been termed centrally mediated abdominal pain syndrome to emphasize the dysregulation of the brain-gut interaction. Once more, alterations in mood and life stressors are associated with the onset of abdominal pain (**Table 12**).

Table 10 Irritable bowel syndrome Rome IV diagnostic criteria and treatment considerations	

Rome IV diagnostic criteria	All of the following for a period of at least 2 mo before diagnosis:
	1. A minimum of 4 d per of abdominal pain associated with one or more of the following:
	   a. Related to defecation
	   b. A change in frequency of stool
	   c. A change in the form or appearance of the stool
	2. In those with constipation, the pain does not resolve with resolution of constipation (if so, this is more consistent with functional constipation)
	3. Symptoms cannot be fully explained by another medical condition

Treatment recommendations	Few double-blind, randomized trials are available to guide treatment • Probiotics • Peppermint oil to reduce severity of pain • Elimination diet to reduce fermentable oligosaccharides, disaccharides, monosaccharides, and polyols • Behavioral treatments to optimize coping skills: hypnotherapy and cognitive behavioral therapy

Adapted from Hyams JS, Di Lorenzo C, Saps M, et al. Childhood functional gastrointestinal disorders: child/adolescent. *Gastroenterology.* 2016;150:1456–68; with permission.

Table 11	
Abdominal migraine Rome IV diagnostic criteria and treatment considerations	

Rome IV diagnostic criteria	All of the following at least twice within 6 mo of diagnosis:
	1. Paroxysmal episodes of intense, acute periumbilical, midline, or diffuse abdominal pain lasting 1 h or longer in duration
	2. Episodes are separated by weeks or months
	3. Pain is incapacitating and interferes with normal activities
	4. Pattern and symptoms are stereotypical in the individual patient
	5. Pain is associated with 2 or more of the following:
	  a. Anorexia
	  b. Nausea
	  c. Vomiting
	  d. Headache
	  e. Photophobia
	  f. Pallor
	6. Symptoms cannot be fully explained by another medical condition

Treatment recommendations	Treatment is determined by frequency, severity, and symptom burden • Rest and sleep • A double-blind, placebo-controlled, crossover trial found benefit for prophylaxis with pizotifen • Additional prophylactic options include amitriptyline, propranolol, and cyproheptadine

Adapted from Hyams JS, Di Lorenzo C, Saps M, et al. Childhood functional gastrointestinal disorders: child/adolescent. *Gastroenterology.* 2016;150:1456–68; with permission.

Table 12	
Functional abdominal pain—not otherwise specified Rome IV diagnostic criteria and treatment considerations	
Rome IV diagnostic criteria	One or more of the following at least 4 times per, for a period of at least 2 mo before diagnosis: 1. Episodic or continuous abdominal pain that does not occur solely during physiologic events (eg, eating, menses) 2. Insufficient criteria for functional dyspepsia, irritable bowel syndrome, or abdominal migraine 3. Symptoms cannot be fully explained by another medical condition
Treatment recommendations	• Hypnotherapy and cognitive behavioral therapy • Citalopram has shown promise compared with placebo • Amitriptyline was effective in a small trial, but a subsequent large multicenter study found a lack of evidence for its use

Adapted from Hyams JS, Di Lorenzo C, Saps M, et al. Childhood functional gastrointestinal disorders: child/adolescent. *Gastroenterology.* 2016;150:1456–68; with permission.

> **Box 1**
> **Red flag signs and symptoms of constipation**
>
> - Passage of meconium for more than 48 hours in a term newborn
> - Constipation in the first month of life
> - Family history of Hirschsprung disease
> - Failure to thrive
> - Bilious vomiting
> - Blood in the stools in the absence of anal fissures
> - Ribbon stools
> - Sacral dimple
> - Tuft of hair on the spine
> - Gluteal cleft deviation
> - Abnormal position of the anus
> - Absent anal or cremasteric reflex
> - Decreased strength/tone/reflexes in the lower extremities
> - Severe abdominal distension
> - Anal scars
>
> *Adapted from* Hyams JS, Di Lorenzo C, Saps M, et al. Childhood functional gastrointestinal disorders: child/adolescent. *Gastroenterology.* 2016;150:1456–68; with permission.

Functional Defecation Disorders

Constipation, and to a lesser degree fecal incontinence, is a common childhood GI complaint; yet, an organic cause of dysregulation in defecation is seldom identifiable. Newborns and toddlers experience anywhere from 4 to 5 bowel movements, or more, per day. However, by the age of 4 years, stools tend to become less numerous, occurring only once to twice per day, and occasionally even more infrequently.[9] Identifying abnormal stooling patterns and navigating the management of these disorders is challenging—estimates reveal that only 50% of patients referred to a tertiary care center for management of constipation were able to successfully wean off of pharmacologic management after 6 to 12 months of follow-up.[9] Likewise, as fecal incontinence possesses a strong correlation with mental and emotional health disturbances, behavioral interventions are necessary to address this issue and require considerable time and effort for effective implementation (**Box 1**).

Functional constipation

Found proportionately among both genders, across socioeconomic classes, and irrespective of dietary practices and cultural influences, functional constipation (FC) is most often elicited by a conscious impulse to avoid defecation, typically due to pain or social situation (travel, school, etc.). Colonic mucosa absorbs water from retained, static feces, causing the stool to become harder and the rectum progressively more distended. Subsequently, this leads to the potential for overflow fecal incontinence, loss of rectal sensation, and worse yet, lack of a normal urge to defecate. Studies estimate an average prevalence of FC at 14% in children.[19] Diagnosis of FC is made by history and physical examination alone; there is no role for the routine use of abdominal radiography in diagnosing FC. That said abdominal radiography may be considered if fecal impaction is suspected in the context of an unreliable physical examination or the clinician is unable to perform an adequate examination. Likewise, laboratory assessment for hypothyroidism, celiac disease, and hypercalcemia are not routinely recommended unless red flag signs or symptoms exist (see later discussion). Barium enema should not be used as a tool for initial evaluation. There is a role for anorectal manometry in children with intractable constipation to evaluate for rectoanal inhibitory reflex (**Table 13**).

Table 13 Functional constipation Rome IV diagnostic criteria and treatment considerations	
Rome IV diagnostic criteria	Two or more of the following occurring at once per week, for a period of at least 1 mo, with insufficient criteria for diagnosis of irritable bowel syndrome: 1. Two or fewer defecations in the toilet per week in a child of developmental age of at least 4 y 2. At least one episode of fecal incontinence per week 3. History of retentive posturing or excessive volitional stool retention 4. History of painful or hard bowel movements 5. Presence of a large fecal mass in the rectum 6. History of large-diameter stools that can obstruct the toilet Symptoms cannot be completely explained by another medical condition
Treatment recommendations	• Behavioral interventions: scheduled toileting, diaries to track stooling, implementation of a rewards system to encourage successful defecation • Polyethylene glycol: first-line pharmacologic agent • Rectal disimpaction if fecal impaction is present

Adapted from Hyams JS, Di Lorenzo C, Saps M, et al. Childhood functional gastrointestinal disorders: child/adolescent. *Gastroenterology.* 2016;150:1456–68; with permission.

Nonretentive fecal incontinence

Nonretentive fecal incontinence (NFI) includes symptoms of uncontrolled defecation without an underlying diagnosis of functional constipation. As many as 4.1% of children in Western societies suffer from NFI.[19] In contrast to FC, children with NFI maintain normal frequency of defecation and exhibit normal GI motility. Sadly, NFI is a common repercussion of prior sexual abuse in children, although it has also been associated with intense fluctuations in emotion. GI transit studies, although not necessary to diagnose this condition, when performed, are normal (**Table 14**).

Table 14	
Nonretentive fecal incontinence Rome IV diagnostic criteria and treatment considerations	
Rome IV diagnostic criteria	One-month history of at least one of the following in a child with developmental age greater than 4 y 1. Defecation into places inappropriate for sociocultural context 2. Lack of evidence of fecal retention 3. Fecal incontinence cannot be explained by another medical condition
Treatment recommendations	• Behavioral therapy: use of rewards, diminishing toilet phobia • Refer victims of prior sexual abuse with nonretentive fecal incontinence to counseling to address psychological disturbances associated with previous trauma

Adapted from Hyams JS, Di Lorenzo C, Saps M, et al. Childhood functional gastrointestinal disorders: child/adolescent. *Gastroenterology*. 2016;150:1456–68; with permission.

REFERENCES

1. Fleisher G. In: Teach SJ, Duryea TK, Wiley F, editors. Approach to diarrhea in children in resource-rich countries. UpToDate; 2019. www.uptodate.com/contents/approach-to-diarrhea-in-children-in-resource-rich-countries?search=infectious%20diarrhea%20children&source=search_result&selectedTitle=2~150&usage_type=default&displa.

2. Crews J. In: Edwards MS, Torchia MM, editors. Clostridioides difficile infection in children: clinical features and diagnosis. UpToDate; 2020. www.uptodate.com/contents/clostridioides-formerly-clostridium-difficile-infection-in-children-clinical-features-and-diagnosis?sectionName=APPROACH%20TO%20DIAGNOSIS&search=infectious%20diarrhea.

3. Kim JH. In: Abrams SA, Kim MS, editors. Neonatal necrotizing enterocolitis: clinical features and diagnosis. UpToDate; 2020. www.uptodate.com/contents/neonatal-necrotizing-enterocolitis-clinical-features-and-diagnosis?search=necrotizing%20enterocolitis&source=search_result&selectedTitle=2~150&usage_type=default&disp.

4. Kim JH. In: Abrams SA, Kim MS, editors. Neonatal necrotizing enterocolitis: management. UpToDate; 2020. www.uptodate.com/contents/neonatal-necrotizing-enterocolitis-management?search=necrotizing%20enterocolitis&source=search_result&selectedTitle=3~150&usage_type=default&display_rank=3.

5. Setty M, et al. In: Motil KJ, Heyman MB, Hoppin AG, editors. Clinical manifestations and complications of inflammatory bowel disease in children and adolescents. UpToDate; 2020. www.uptodate.com/contents/clinical-manifestations-and-complications-of-inflammatory-bowel-disease-in-children-and-adolescents?search=inflammatory%20bowel%20disease%20children&source=search_res.

6. Higuchi LM, Bousvaros A. In: Heyman MB, Hoppin AG, editors. Clinical presentation and diagnosis of inflammatory bowel disease in children. UpToDate; 2020. www.uptodate.com/contents/clinical-presentation-and-diagnosis-of-inflammatory-

bowel-disease-in-children?search=inflammatory%20bowel%20disease%20children&source=search_result&selectedTitle=1~15.

7. Zitomersky N, Bousvaros A. In: Motil KJ, Heyman MB, Hoppin AG, editors. Overview of the management of Crohn disease in children and adolescents. UpToDate; 2020. https://www.uptodate.com/contents/overview-of-the-management-of-crohn-disease-in-children-and-adolescents?search=inflammatory%20bowel%20disease%20children&sectionRank=2&usage_type=default&anchor=H824 1845&source=machineLearning&selectedTitle=5~150&display_rank=5#H824 1845.

8. Vandenplas Y, Brueton M, Dupont C, et al. Guidelines for the diagnosis and management of cow's milk protein allergy in infants. Arch Dis Child 2007;92:902–8.

9. Brown LJ, Miller LT. Pediatrics. Baltimore: Lippincoot Williams & Wilkins; 2005. p. 283–323.

10. Wesson DE, Lopez ME. In: Singer JI, Li BU, Hoppin AG, editors. Congenital aganglionic megacolon (Hirschsprung disease). UpToDate; 2019. www.uptodate.com/contents/congenital-aganglionic-megacolon-hirschsprung-disease?search=hirschsprung&source=search_result&selectedTitle=1~79&usage_type=default&display_rank=1.

11. Olive AP, Endom EE. In: Singer JI, Li BU, Hoppin AG, editors. Infantile hypertrophic pyloric stenosis. UpToDate; 2020. www.uptodate.com/contents/infantile-hypertrophic-pyloric-stenosis?search=pyloric%20stenosis&source=search_result&selectedTitle=1~77&usage_type=default&display_rank=1.

12. Wilson CM, Evans JS, Kay MH. Functional gastrointestinal disorders in pediatric and adolescent patients. American College of Gastroenterology; 2013. gi.org/topics/functional-gastrointestinal-disorders-in-pediatric-and-adolescent-patients/.

13. Hambidge SJ, Davidson AJ, Gonzales R, et al. Epidemiology of pediatric injury-related primary care office visits in the United States. Pediatrics 2002;109(4):559–65.

14. McOmber MA, Shulman RJ. Pediatric functional gastrointestinal disorders. Nutr Clin Pract 2008;23(3):268–74.

15. Puntis JW. Childhood disease: gastrointestinal problems. Pharm J 2000;144. gi.org/topics/functional-gastrointestinal-disorders-in-pediatric-and-adolescent-patients/.

16. Boston Children's Hospital. Functional abdominal pain in children. www.childrenshospital.org/conditions-and-treatments/conditions/f/functional-abdominal-pain#:~:text=Functional%20abdominal%20pain%2C%20also%20known,abdominal%20pain%20at%20some%20point. Accessed October 11, 2020.

17. Oudenhove LV, Crowell MD, Drossman DA, et al. Biopsychosocial aspects of functional gastrointestinal disorders: how central and environmental processes contribute to the development and expression of functional gastrointestinal disorders. Gastroenterology 2016;150:1355–67.

18. Drossman, Douglas A. Functional gastrointestinal disorders: history, pathophysiology, clinical features, and rome IV. Gastroenterology 2016;150:1262–79.

19. Hyams JS, Lorenzo CD, Saps M, et al. Childhood functional gastrointestinal disorders: child/adolescent. Gastroenterology 2016;150:1456–68.

20. Irritable Bowel Syndrome. Boston Children's Hospital. https://www.childrenshospital.org/conditions-and-treatments/conditions/i/ibs. Accessed October 11, 2020.

Autism Spectrum Disorders

Ashley Iles, MD

KEYWORDS

• Autism • Spectrum disorders • Asperger • Primary care • Pediatrics

KEY POINTS

- The prevalence of autistic spectrum disorders (ASDs) appears to be increasing year to year in the US population.
- Developmental screening for all pediatric patients is recommended, and specific ASD screening tools are available.
- The etiology of ASD is complex and multifactorial involving genetics, neurobiologic changes, and environmental exposures leading to a heterogeneous presentation of behaviors.
- Treatment for ASD should involve specialists familiar with these disorders and, if possible, a multidisciplinary team to provide comprehensive medical and social support for the patient and family.
- Significantly more research is needed to determine optimal treatment strategies and outcome measures for patients with ASD.

HISTORY AND BACKGROUND

The condition of autism was first described in the 1940s. Both Leo Kanner and Hans Asperger began publishing on the condition almost simultaneously.[1,2] It had long been thought to be a coincidence, but more recent publications suggest there may have been a connection between their work.[3] In the decades since, classifications of autism and its related disorders have continued to evolve. Most recently, the American Psychiatric Association has combined previously distinct diagnoses under the broader diagnosis of autism spectrum disorder (ASD) in their *Diagnostic and Statistical Manual of Mental Disorders, Fifth Edition* (DSM-5).[4] Previous disorders from their fourth edition (DSM-IV) that now fall under this category include autistic disorders, Asperger syndrome, and pervasive developmental disorder.[4] The condition itself is now recognized as a heterogeneous spectrum of social communication deficits and repetitive sensory-motor behaviors that can range from mildly to severely debilitating.[5] Awareness and advocacy have improved in especially significant ways since the turn of the century. The organization Autism Speaks, founded in 2005, has heavily focused on global advocacy with much success. In 2007, the United Nations instituted the World Autism Awareness Day, celebrated annually on April 2.

215 Central Avenue Suite 100, Louisville, KY 40208, USA
E-mail address: ashley.iles@louisville.edu

Prim Care Clin Office Pract 48 (2021) 461–473
https://doi.org/10.1016/j.pop.2021.04.003
0095-4543/21/© 2021 Elsevier Inc. All rights reserved.

PREVALENCE

Because there are challenges related to the diagnosis of ASD, data reporting on the presence of it in a population depends almost exclusively on prevalence data, rather than incidence or other more precise measures. Accurate data are difficult to obtain, as the definitions, diagnostic practices, and even lack of awareness have obstructed the study of autism disorders over the past century.[6,7]

Increasing Prevalence

Since the earliest prevalence data were reported until now, there has been concern about a significant prevalence increase over time.[7] Some studies have indicated an increase from as many as 4 cases per 10,000 people to 60 cases per 10,000 people.[7,8] Much has been written on this topic over the past 2 decades attempting to identify reasons for the reported increase.[7–9] There is no doubt that some of the difference comes from changes in diagnostic criteria and practice. For example, one study done in California demonstrated that diagnostic criteria changes could account for up to one-quarter of the observed increase in autism diagnoses between 1992 and 2005.[10] At least 1 study, attempting to estimate the global burden of disease for ASD, concluded there was no clear evidence for a change in prevalence between 1990 and 2010.[11] As mentioned previously, there was an update to the classification of pervasive developmental disorder (PDD) in DSM-IV published in 1994, now included as part of the autism spectrum disorders named by the DSM-5 published in 2013. Because it has been demonstrated that many patients meet criteria for ASD per the DSM-5 guidelines that did not previously,[12,13] it is reasonable to conclude that diagnostic changes contribute to the increases seen in prevalence more recently, although the full extent of this effect is admittedly uncertain.

Fortunately, as awareness, screening strategies, and standardization of diagnostic criteria improve, so does our confidence in the accuracy of current prevalence. In 2000, the Centers for Disease Control and Prevention put together a surveillance network, Autism and Developmental Disabilities Monitoring Network, encompassing 11 different sites to monitor the prevalence of ASD in the US population. Their data are continually updated and reported providing much needed insight into the pervasiveness of the disorders, as well as the potential impacts for the United States. For 2016, ASD prevalence was 18.5 per 1000 (1 in 54) children aged 8 years averaged across all 11 sites.[14] In the same year, a national parental survey demonstrated similar prevalence in children ages 3 to 17, approximately 1 in 40.[15] This does represent an increase from that reported in 2012, when the prevalence was 14.5 per 1000 (1 in 69) across the 11 sites.[16] Additional observation will be needed to determine the stability of the prevalence over time.

Additional Trends

Other statistical trends have been well established, including that of the consistently higher rates of ASD in male over female individuals.[17] This disproportionate effect is evident in the ADDM network data, as ASD was 4.3 times more prevalent in boys over girls in the 2016 data[14] and 4.5 times in the 2012 data.[16] Some analysis has suggested that the ratio may be closer to 3:1 overall male-to-female.[17] Other trends in the data including those seen in race/ethnicity are conflicting and likely confounded by data collection techniques, socioeconomic differences, and other factors.[14,16] Finally, global data may suggest a similar prevalence across industrialized countries,[11] but much more data are needed in especially low-income and middle-income countries to determine the impact of disease.[6]

ETIOLOGY AND RISK FACTORS

The search for the cause of ASD has led researchers down many pathways. Our current understanding of the etiology of disease is incomplete, but genetic factors, environmental exposures, and maternal/perinatal risk factors have all been implicated in the behavioral and neurobiological manifestations of disease.[5,18,19]

Risk Factors

Table 1 summarizes many of the investigated risk factors associated with ASD. It is important to note that causation for any one of these factors has not been established, although there have been many theories suggested regarding how they might contribute to the disruption of neurodevelopment.

In addition to these, maternal use of selective serotonin reuptake inhibitors (SSRIs) has been an area of research, but studies have suggested the association may be related to the presence of psychiatric disease in the mother rather than an exposure to the medications themselves.[24,25] Other studies have looked at an entity called "endocrine-disrupting chemicals" without a definitive association yet made.[20,26]

Much more research in the area of exposures is still needed to provide clarity. However, it is unlikely that a single risk factor or exposure is responsible for the increased prevalence of ASD over time.

Protective Factors

Several factors have been proposed as possibly decreasing risk of ASD. However, it is challenging to distinguish general developmental protective factors from those specific to ASD. Folate supplementation has been one suggested protective factor, but there is some conflicting evidence about its association with rates of ASD traits and also some evidence that very high levels may increase ASD risk.[18,23] Other potential, but yet unproven protective factors may include adequate breastfeeding, iron supplementation, and multivitamin supplementation.[23]

Genetics

The heritable nature of ASD has been well-demonstrated through family and twin studies.[27] The exact proportion of contribution from heritable versus nonheritable

Table 1	
Autism spectrum disorder risk factors	
Categories	**Specific Risks**
Maternal factors[5,18–20]	• Advanced maternal age • Obesity, diabetes mellitus, hypertension • Short pregnancy intervals (<12–24 mo) • Hospitalization for infection during pregnancy • Maternal/familial autoimmune disease history
Perinatal/Neonatal factors[20,21]	• Abnormal/breech presentation • Umbilical cord complications • Fetal distress • Multiple births • Low birth weight/small for gestational age • Congenital malformations • Hyperbilirubinemia
Environmental factors[18,20,22,23]	• Particulate matter • Valproate exposure

factors is still up for debate.[5,19,28] Improved technologies have contributed to more specific examinations of the genetic origins of ASD and the development of clinical applications for genetic testing. The genetic contributions are quite complex and demonstrate genetic and phenotypic heterogeneity that favors a complex inheritance pattern involving many variants.[5,18] Although the American Academy of Pediatrics (AAP) does recommend a thorough etiologic workup including genetic testing, such testing should be done by a provider/specialist with the knowledge and expertise to interpret the findings and advise families regarding the clinical implications of the results.[19]

Neurobiology

Certain neurobiologic patterns are associated with ASD. One such pattern is decreased brain volume at certain stages of early development.[29] There is other evidence that suggests lower connectivity in the brain systems is also present in patients with ASD.[30] Although we know that these neuroanatomic changes exist, many biomarkers for disease have been studied and none to date have demonstrated reliability for diagnostic purposes thus far.[29,31] Similarly, genetic testing can potentially provide some insights into etiology for specific cases of ASD, but the presence of any particular genetic finding does not guarantee the presence of phenotypic autistic behaviors.[5] Therefore, the diagnostic criteria remain in the realm of observable behaviors for the present (see Diagnosis).

SCREENINGS

Current Recommendations

The AAP recommends screening of all children at ages 18 months and 24 months with the most validated tools available.[19] The US Preventive Services Task Force (USPSTF) position statement is different, placing autism screening in the "I" category, citing insufficient evidence of improved outcomes for screening the general population.[32] It would be incorrect to use their recommendation as a reason to not perform screening in primary care, as they clarify, "In the absence of evidence about the balance of benefits and harms, clinicians should use their clinical judgment to decide if screening in children without overt signs and symptoms is appropriate for the population in their care."[32]

Limitations

Several investigators have attempted to offer insights into the validity and reliability of screening tools currently available, of which there are more than 30.[33,34] Challenges to screening include the following: expected behavioral differences across age groups, changing diagnostic criteria, and accessibility of screening tools.[33] The effects of ethnicity and culture on the screening outcomes need to be considered.[35] In addition, the signs and symptoms used in screening tools for ASD overlap with other neurodevelopmental disorders.[33] It is also worth noting that most screening tools were developed before the publication of the updated DSM-5 in 2013. Further research and development are needed to address these gaps and to answer the question of whether screening has demonstrable effects on patient outcomes.[32,33]

Screening Tools

Despite these limitations, screening tools may assist clinical practice, and more appear to be in development. Of these, the most commonly used and well-studied is the Modified Checklist for Autism in Toddlers (MCHAT), which has gone through several cycles of modification with the most recent version being the MCHAT,

Revised, with Follow-up (MCHAT-R/F). It has an approximate positive predictive value of 50%[36,37] and is available for free download for use in clinical, research, and educational purposes. It is subject to some of the limitations previously discussed, including a limited age range of applicability of 18 to 24 months. Even within that range, some believe the screening may need to differ as the developmental milestones (especially in language) are quite different between 18 and 24 months.[38] However, both the AAP and USPSTF deem it acceptable for current widespread use.[19,32]

The MCHAT-R/F is called such because it is set up as a 2-step screen. If a patient screens positive on the MCHAT-R, the follow-up questions are provided to further evaluate for false positives (of which they admit the rate is relatively high). Any patient who ultimately screens positive should be referred for a more detailed evaluation by a specialist.[19] In addition, if a parent reports concerns or concerning behavior is witnessed by a provider, further investigation is always warranted regardless of the general screening recommendations.[19,32] Many additional tools for evaluation of patients (in other age groups, for example) exist and may be used, but a detailed discussion of these is outside the scope of this article.[33]

DIAGNOSIS

Some of the earliest signs of ASD may appear within the first year of life,[39] but accurate diagnosis typically requires the observation of behaviors over time. The qualifying criteria are described in detail by the DSM-5. The core requirements are detailed in **Box 1**. To meet the requirements of diagnosis, the patient must have deficits in 2 domains, social and behavioral, as well as symptoms present early on in development that cause significant impairment.

Social Impairments

The social impairments indicative of the disorder include communication and interaction deficits. The DSM-5 describes 3 manifestations of these that are present in the disorder, although more may be present as well. First, patients demonstrate social-emotional reciprocity deficits such that they either do not respond in socially appropriate ways or are unable to respond or initiate such interactions altogether. This includes a reduced ability to share emotions, interests, or affect.[4]

Second, patients will demonstrate a deficit in nonverbal communication behaviors, such that their nonverbal communication is either abnormal or absent. Nonverbal communication such as eye movements, hand gestures, and facial expressions might be poorly integrated, inappropriately applied, or absent altogether.[4]

Third, impairments will be present in the development, maintenance, and understanding of relationships. These patients will not be able to adapt well to differing social contexts, and they may struggle to form social relationships or demonstrate no interest in peer interactions.[4]

Box 1
Diagnostic criteria for autism spectrum disorder[4]

1. Social communication and social interaction deficits
   a. Persistent
   b. Present in multiple contexts

2. Restricted, repetitive patterns of behavior, interests, or activities

3. Symptoms are present in the early developmental period

4. Symptoms cause significant impairment

Behavioral Abnormalities

Abnormal behaviors associated with ASD are described as restrictive and repetitive. **Table 2** details examples of these behaviors. Per the DSM-5, the presence of at least 2 of the patterns of behavior are required for diagnosis of ASD.

In the DSM-5, there are also criteria for classifying the level of severity given the significant heterogeneity of presentations in patients with ASD. Level 1 is classified as patients "requiring support" citing noticeable impairments in function but in the presence of intact communication abilities; in contrast to the highest Level 3 patients who "require very substantial support" and who have severe deficits in both verbal and nonverbal communication skills, as well as restrictive or repetitive behaviors that impair function in all spheres. The criteria themselves are somewhat ambiguous and not quantifiable for tracking disease progress, but may be helpful in qualifying patients who need especially high levels of interventions, social services, and support.[4,19]

CONSIDERATIONS

Associated Conditions

ASD is an independent diagnosis based on the criteria described, but it is often associated with other conditions, impairments, and symptoms that contribute to the complexity of caring for and treating these patients. Patients with ASD have high rates of other psychiatric disorders, anywhere from 50% to 90%.[40–42] Some of the most commonly identified include anxiety disorders, depression, attention-deficit/hyperactivity disorder (ADHD), oppositional defiant disorder, obsessive compulsive disorder, and schizophrenia.[40–44] Of these, anxiety disorders appear to be the most common.

In addition, sleep disorders are very common, occurring at rates as high as 50% to 80%.[45,46] Epilepsy occurs at higher rates in patients with ASD than in the general population,[47] and gastrointestinal symptoms are more common, including chronic constipation and diarrhea.[48,49] There is some evidence that other chronic diseases such as hypertension, diabetes, dyslipidemia, and obesity are also present at significantly higher rates in patients with ASD.[44] All of these contribute to the challenge of medically caring for patients with ASD, especially when the ASD symptoms or intellectual disabilities inhibit the patient from communicating their symptoms.

Table 2
Typical behavior patterns in autism spectrum disorder[4]

Pattern Type:	Examples:
Repetitive motor movements, use of objects, or speech	*Lining up of toys, flipping objects, parroting of another's spoken words, hand flapping, finger flicking*
Strong preference for sameness, adherence to routines, or ritualized behavior patterns	*Distress with change, difficulty with transitions, strict rule adherence, repetitive questioning, perimeter pacing*
Restricted, fixated interests abnormal in intensity or focus	*Strong attachment to particular object (children), preoccupation with a particular type of object, excessive time diagramming a topic (adult)*
Hyperactivity or hyporeactivity to sensory input or unusual interest in sensory aspects of the environment	*Extreme responses to certain sounds or smells, preoccupation with lights or moving objects, indifference to pain or temperature*

Outcomes

Among patients with the diagnosis of ASD, there is a significant variability in the level of impairment each patient experiences across various domains (eg, intellectual disability, verbal IQ). Predicting the eventual level of impairment at time of diagnosis in early childhood is not possible, and there is much inconsistency in how outcomes are evaluated and reported.[50] Diagnostic rates appear to be stable over time (once diagnosed, a patient will continue to carry the diagnosis), but other outcome measures need significantly more study.[51] Not surprisingly, patients with ASD have poorer outcomes than their peers in the realms of employment, relationships, independent living, and mental health.[50] The factors that do improve outcomes based on current evidence are those involving social support and inclusion practices.[52,53]

THERAPEUTIC OPTIONS

There is a general consensus that the appropriate management of patients with ASD involves a multidisciplinary approach in light of the heterogeneity of impairments, severity, comorbid conditions, and social supports needed.[5,19,54] Providing and coordinating such care is challenging, and much discussion exists around improving its coordination and the pathways to optimal care for these patients and families.[54–56] The approach to therapy should be comprehensive, designed to address broad goals for the patient in terms of improved behavior and function, referred to as "comprehensive treatment models" (CTM).[57] If preestablished pathways to CTMs and multidisciplinary treatment teams exist in the local health care system, they should be used and every effort made by primary care providers to connect patients to the appropriate services.

Behavioral Therapies

Many therapy paradigms have been developed over time under different names, but many of them have overlapping principles and treatment elements.[60] The development of these techniques started in the 1960s and most treatment paradigms are grounded in the principles of applied behavioral analysis (ABA).[58] More recently, approaches called "naturalistic developmental behavioral interventions" have made use of ABA principles, but incorporate the use of natural environments and feedback techniques with encouraging results.[59,60] The varied schemes and intervention labels, along with inconsistent evaluation methods, contributes to the difficulties in obtaining quality evidence in the study of efficacy for these interventions.[61,62] However, these techniques continue to be the mainstay of treatment for patients with ASD.

In addition to the central therapy techniques, many adjunctive therapies have been studied over time. Some that include decent evidence of benefit include parental instruction,[63] music therapy,[64] physical activity,[65,66] and equine therapy.[67,68] These types of therapies may be more useful for particular domains of impairment, rather than broadly beneficial. However, more research will need to be done to make specific claims of efficacy.

Medications

There is no comprehensive or universally recommended medication regimen for patients with ASD. Typically, medications are viewed as an adjunct way to address particular problematic behaviors and/or comorbid conditions. **Table 3** lists a few of the most commonly used medications in these patients.

The atypical antipsychotics aripiprazole and risperidone are the current Food and Drug Administration (FDA)-approved medications used to address ASD-related irritability, which can include behaviors such as agitation, self-injurious behavior, and

Table 3		
Medications commonly used in autism spectrum disorders		
Indication	Medication	Comments
Irritability	Aripiprazole, risperidone[69]	Both FDA approved for this purpose
Sleep disturbance	Melatonin[70]	
ADHD	Methylphenidate, atomoxetine, guanfacine, clonidine[71,72]	Methylphenidate has some established efficacy[72] Other medications are undergoing additional study
Mood disorders	More investigation needed	SSRIs have mixed evidence in these patients[19,71,73] Other medications under study include SNRIs and buspirone.

Abbreviations: ADHD, attention-deficit/hyperactivity disorder; FDA, Food and Drug Administration; SNRI, serotonin-norepinephrine reuptake inhibitor; SSRI, selective serotonin reuptake inhibitor.

tantrums/outbursts.[69] The efficacy of these medications is relatively well established for such behaviors,[69,74,75] but may also benefit in other behavior realms.[19] Unfortunately, the possible side effects of these medications are extensive and include extrapyramidal symptoms. The most common appear to be increased appetite and weight gain.[76] There is some evidence that relapse rates to aggressive behaviors are equivocal between aripiprazole and placebo.[74] Therefore, once a patient is stabilized, reevaluation of use of these medications may be warranted, especially when adequate behavioral therapy strategies are implemented.

Many other medications have been studied in ASD to assist with other comorbid conditions or difficult-to-control symptoms. For cocurrent ADHD symptoms, methylphenidate has some evidence of efficacy,[71,72] and others that have been used include clonidine, guanfacine, and atomoxetine. For symptoms of poor sleep, efficacious interventions may include melatonin, but behavioral intervention and parent education as well.[70] Other forms of nutritional supplementation have been proposed for use addressing various symptoms associated with ASD, but there is poor evidence for any of one them at this time and there are potential risks of toxicity with high-dose supplementation approaches.[77]

Unfortunately, mood disturbances in patients with ASD remain difficult to treat without clear efficacy for any one medication or class in all patients. The evidence for use of SSRIs is mixed,[73] and further investigation into other potential options including buspirone is needed.[71] The challenges of medical intervention in these patients reinforces the appropriateness of specialist referral to assist with management.

SUMMARY

For the primary care practitioner, the focus on ASD should consist of early identification of abnormal development/behaviors and early referral to specialists for further evaluation and targeted treatment. It is important to be familiar with resources available to patients, parents, and families in the local context. However, given the paucity of specialists in some geographic areas, primary care providers should strive to have a fundamental understanding of ASD and the basic medical interventions to comanage care as needed. Significantly more research is needed on numerous aspects of these disorders to improve clinical care and outcomes for patients.

CLINICS CARE POINTS

- Signs and behaviors associated with ASD may appear as early as the first year of life.
- The AAP recommends that all patients be screened for ASD with the most optimal screening test available, typically at 18 and 24 months of age.
- The diagnostic criteria for ASD have been updated with the publication of the DSM-5 by the American Psychiatric Association in 2013 to include the previously separate diagnoses of PDD and Asperger syndrome.
- Although medications may have some utility in treating aspects of problematic behaviors, the mainstay of ASD treatment is behavioral therapy.
- ADHD, anxiety disorders, and other psychiatric conditions are frequently diagnosed as comorbid conditions in patients with ASD.

DISCLOSURE

No disclosures or conflicts.

REFERENCES

1. Kanner L. Autistic disturbances of affective contact 1943.
2. Asperger H. Die "Autistischen Psychopathen" im Kindesalter. Archiv F Psychiatrie 1944;117:76–136.
3. Chown N, Hughes L. History and first descriptions of autism: Asperger versus Kanner revisited. J Autism Dev Disord 2016;46(6):2270–2.
4. American Psychiatric Association. Neurodevelopmental Disorders, Diagnostic and statistical Manual of mental disorders: DSM-5. 5th edition. Arlington, VA: American Psychiatric Association; 2013.
5. Lord C, Elsabbagh M, Baird G, et al. Autism spectrum disorder. Lancet 2018; 392(10146):508–20.
6. Elsabbagh M, Divan G, Koh YJ, et al. Global prevalence of autism and other pervasive developmental disorders. Autism Res 2012;5(3):160–79.
7. Rutter M. Incidence of autism spectrum disorders: changes over time and their meaning. Acta Paediatr 2005;94(1):2–15.
8. Wing L, Potter D. The epidemiology of autistic spectrum disorders: is the prevalence rising? Ment Retard Dev Disabil Res Rev 2002;8(3):151–61.
9. Fombonne E. Editorial: the rising prevalence of autism. J Child Psychol Psychiatry 2018;59(7):717–20.
10. King M, Bearman P. Diagnostic change and the increased prevalence of autism. Int J Epidemiol 2009;38(5):1224–34.
11. Baxter AJ, Brugha TS, Erskine HE, et al. The epidemiology and global burden of autism spectrum disorders. Psychol Med 2015;45(3):601–13.
12. Bishop DV, Whitehouse AJ, Watt HJ, et al. Autism and diagnostic substitution: evidence from a study of adults with a history of developmental language disorder. Dev Med Child Neurol 2008;50(5):341–5.
13. Kim YS, Fombonne E, Koh YJ, et al. A comparison of DSM-IV pervasive developmental disorder and DSM-5 autism spectrum disorder prevalence in an epidemiologic sample. J Am Acad Child Adolesc Psychiatry 2014;53(5):500–8.
14. Maenner MJ, Shaw KA, Baio J, et al. Prevalence of autism spectrum disorder among children aged 8 years — autism and developmental disabilities monitoring network, 11 sites, United States, 2016. MMWR Surveill Summ 2020;69:1–12.

15. Kogan MD, Vladutiu CJ, Schieve LA, et al. The prevalence of parent-reported autism spectrum disorder among US children. Pediatrics 2018;142(6):1–11.

16. Christensen DL, Braun KVN, Baio J, et al. Prevalence and characteristics of autism spectrum disorder among children aged 8 years - Autism and developmental disabilities monitoring network, 11 sites, United States, 2012. MMWR Surveill Summ 2018;65(13):1–23.

17. Loomes R, Hull L, Mandy WPL. What is the male-to-female ratio in autism spectrum disorder? A systematic review and meta-analysis. J Am Acad Child Adolesc Psychiatry 2017;56(6):466–74.

18. Lyall K, Croen L, Daniels J, et al. The changing epidemiology of autism spectrum disorders. Annu Rev Public Health 2017;38:81–102.

19. Hyman SL, Levy SE, Myers SM. Identification, evaluation, and management of children with autism spectrum disorder. Pediatrics 2020;145(1):e20193447.

20. Modabbernia A, Velthorst E, Reichenberg A. Environmental risk factors for autism: an evidence-based review of systematic reviews and meta-analyses. Mol Autism 2017;8:13.

21. Gardener H, Spiegelman D, Buka SL. Perinatal and neonatal risk factors for autism: a comprehensive meta-analysis. Pediatrics 2011;128(2):344–55.

22. Christensen J, Grønborg TK, Sørensen MJ, et al. Prenatal valproate exposure and risk of autism spectrum disorders and childhood autism. JAMA 2013;309(16): 1696–703.

23. Cheng J, Eskenazi B, Widjaja F, et al. Improving autism perinatal risk factors: a systematic review. Med Hypotheses 2019;127:26–33.

24. Kaplan YC, Keskin-Arslan E, Acar S, et al. Maternal SSRI discontinuation, use, psychiatric disorder and the risk of autism in children: a meta-analysis of cohort studies. Br J Clin Pharmacol 2017;83(12):2798–806.

25. Kim JY, Son MJ, Son CY, et al. Environmental risk factors and biomarkers for autism spectrum disorder: an umbrella review of the evidence. Lancet Psychiatry 2019;6(7):590–600.

26. Moosa A, Shu H, Sarachana T, et al. Are endocrine disrupting compounds environmental risk factors for autism spectrum disorder? Horm Behav 2018;101: 13–21.

27. Sandin S, Lichtenstein P, Kuja-Halkola R, et al. The familial risk of autism. JAMA 2014;311(17):1770–7.

28. Sanchack KE, Thomas CA. Autism spectrum disorder: primary care principles. Am Fam Physician 2016;94(12):972–9.

29. Ecker C, Bookheimer SY, Murphy DG. Neuroimaging in autism spectrum disorder: brain structure and function across the lifespan. Lancet Neurol 2015; 14(11):1121–34.

30. Rane P, Cochran D, Hodge SM, et al. Connectivity in autism: a review of MRI connectivity studies. Harv Rev Psychiatry 2015;23:223–44.

31. Uddin LQ, Dajani DR, Voorhies W, et al. Progress and roadblocks in the search for brain-based biomarkers of autism and attention-deficit/hyperactivity disorder. Transl Psychiatry 2017;7(8):e1218.

32. Siu AL, Bibbins-Domingo K, Grossman DC, et al. Screening for autism spectrum disorder in young children: US preventive services task force recommendation statement. JAMA 2016;315(7):691–6.

33. Thabtah F, Peebles D. Early autism screening: a comprehensive review. Int J Environ Res Public Health 2019;16(18):3502.

34. Sánchez-García AB, Galindo-Villardón P, Nieto-Librero AB, et al. Toddler screening for autism spectrum disorder: a meta-analysis of diagnostic accuracy. J Autism Dev Disord 2019;49(5):1837–52.
35. Rea KE, Armstrong-Brine M, Ramirez L, et al. Ethnic disparities in autism spectrum disorder screening and referral: implications for pediatric practice. J Dev Behav Pediatr 2019;40(7):493–500.
36. Robins DL, Casagrande K, Barton M, et al. Validation of the modified checklist for autism in toddlers, revised with follow-up (M-CHAT-R/F). Pediatrics 2014;133(1): 37–45.
37. Chlebowski C, Robins DL, Barton ML, et al. Large-scale use of the modified checklist for autism in low-risk toddlers. Pediatrics 2013;131(4):e1121–7.
38. Sturner R, Howard B, Bergmann P, et al. Accurate autism screening at the 18-month well-child visit requires different strategies than at 24 months. J Autism Dev Disord 2017;47(10):3296–310.
39. Zwaigenbaum L, Bryson S, Rogers T, et al. Behavioral manifestations of autism in the first year of life. Int J Dev Neurosci 2005;23(2–3):143–52.
40. Buck TR, Viskochil J, Farley M, et al. Psychiatric comorbidity and medication use in adults with autism spectrum disorder. J Autism Dev Disord 2014;44(12): 3063–71.
41. Salazar F, Baird G, Chandler S, et al. Co-occurring psychiatric disorders in preschool and elementary school-aged children with autism spectrum disorder. J Autism Dev Disord 2015;45(8):2283–94.
42. Simonoff E, Pickles A, Charman T, et al. Psychiatric disorders in children with autism spectrum disorders: prevalence, comorbidity, and associated factors in a population-derived sample. J Am Acad Child Adolesc Psychiatry 2008;47(8): 921–9.
43. Bakken TL, Helverschou SB, Eilertsen DE, et al. Psychiatric disorders in adolescents and adults with autism and intellectual disability: a representative study in one county in Norway. Res Dev Disabil 2010;31(6):1669–77.
44. Croen LA, Zerbo O, Qian Y, et al. The health status of adults on the autism spectrum. Autism 2015;19(7):814–23.
45. Singh K, Zimmerman AW. Sleep in autism spectrum disorder and attention deficit hyperactivity disorder. Semin Pediatr Neurol 2015;22(2):113–25.
46. Robinson-Shelton A, Malow BA. Sleep disturbances in neurodevelopmental disorders. Curr Psychiatry Rep 2016;18(1):6.
47. Lukmanji S, Manji SA, Kadhim S, et al. The co-occurrence of epilepsy and autism: a systematic review. Epilepsy Behav 2019;98:238–48.
48. Holingue C, Newill C, Lee LC, et al. Gastrointestinal symptoms in autism spectrum disorder: a review of the literature on ascertainment and prevalence. Autism Res 2018;11(1):24–36.
49. Lefter R, Ciobica A, Timofte D, et al. A descriptive review on the prevalence of gastrointestinal disturbances and their multiple associations in autism spectrum disorder. Medicina 2019;56(1):11.
50. Howlin P, Magiati I. Autism spectrum disorder: outcomes in adulthood. Curr Opin Psychiatry 2017;30(2):69–76.
51. Magiati I, Tay XW, Howlin P. Cognitive, language, social and behavioural outcomes in adults with autism spectrum disorders: a systematic review of longitudinal follow-up studies in adulthood. Clin Psychol Rev 2014;34(1):73–86.
52. Renty JO, Roeyers H. Quality of life in high-functioning adults with autism spectrum disorder: the predictive value of disability and support characteristics. Autism 2006;10(5):511–24.

53. Woodman AC, Smith LE, Greenberg JS, et al. Contextual factors predict patterns of change in functioning over 10 years among adolescents and adults with autism spectrum disorders. J Autism Dev Disord 2016;46(1):176–89.
54. Thom RP, McDougle CJ, Hazen EP. Challenges in the medical care of patients with autism spectrum disorder: the role of the consultation-liaison psychiatrist. Psychosomatics 2019;60(5):435–43.
55. Hurt L, Langley K, North K, et al. Understanding and improving the care pathway for children with autism. Int J Health Care Qual Assur 2019;32(1):208–23.
56. Austin J, Manning-Courtney P, Johnson ML, et al. Improving access to care at autism treatment centers: a system analysis approach. Pediatrics 2016;137: 149–57.
57. Wong C, Odom SL, Hume KA, et al. Evidence-based practices for children, youth, and young adults with autism spectrum disorder: a comprehensive review. J Autism Dev Disord 2015;45(7):1951–66.
58. Schreibman L, Dawson G, Stahmer AC, et al. Naturalistic developmental behavioral interventions: empirically validated treatments for autism spectrum disorder. J Autism Dev Disord 2015;45(8):2411–28.
59. Sandbank M, Bottema-Beutel K, Crowley S, et al. Project AIM: autism intervention meta-analysis for studies of young children. Psychol Bull 2020;146(1):1–29.
60. Tiede G, Walton KM. Meta-analysis of naturalistic developmental behavioral interventions for young children with autism spectrum disorder. Autism 2019;23(8): 2080–95.
61. French L, Kennedy EMM. Annual research review: early intervention for infants and young children with, or at-risk of, autism spectrum disorder: a systematic review. J Child Psychol Psychiatry 2018;59(4):444–56.
62. Vivanti G, Kasari C, Green J, et al. Implementing and evaluating early intervention for children with autism: where are the gaps and what should we do? Autism Res 2018;11(1):16–23.
63. Bradshaw J, Bearss K, McCracken C, et al. Parent education for young children with autism and disruptive behavior: response to active control treatment. J Clin Child Adolesc Psychol 2018;47:S445–55.
64. Geretsegger M, Elefant C, Mössler KA, et al. Music therapy for people with autism spectrum disorder. Cochrane Database Syst Rev 2014;2014(6):CD004381.
65. Howells K, Sivaratnam C, May T, et al. Efficacy of group-based organised physical activity participation for social outcomes in children with autism spectrum disorder: a systematic review and meta-analysis. J Autism Dev Disord 2019;49(8): 3290–308.
66. Tan BW, Pooley JA, Speelman CP. A meta-analytic review of the efficacy of physical exercise interventions on cognition in individuals with autism spectrum disorder and ADHD. J Autism Dev Disord 2016;46(9):3126–43.
67. Srinivasan SM, Cavagnino DT, Bhat AN. Effects of equine therapy on individuals with autism spectrum disorder: a systematic review. Rev J Autism Dev Disord 2018;5(2):156–75.
68. McDaniel Peters BC, Wood W. Autism and equine-assisted interventions: a systematic mapping review. J Autism Dev Disord 2017;47(10):3220–42.
69. Fung LK, Mahajan R, Nozzolillo A, et al. Pharmacologic treatment of severe irritability and problem behaviors in autism: a systematic review and meta-analysis. Pediatrics 2016;137:S124–35.
70. Cuomo BM, Vaz S, Lee EAL, et al. Effectiveness of sleep-based interventions for children with autism spectrum disorder: a meta-synthesis. Pharmacotherapy 2017;37(5):555–78.

71. Goel R, Hong JS, Findling RL, et al. An update on pharmacotherapy of autism spectrum disorder in children and adolescents. Int Rev Psychiatry 2018;30(1): 78–95.
72. Sturman N, Deckx L, van Driel ML. Methylphenidate for children and adolescents with autism spectrum disorder. Cochrane Database Syst Rev 2017;11(11): CD011144.
73. Williams K, Brignell A, Randall M, et al. Selective serotonin reuptake inhibitors (SSRIs) for autism spectrum disorders (ASD). Cochrane Database Syst Rev 2013;8:CD004677.
74. Hirsch LE, Pringsheim T. Aripiprazole for autism spectrum disorders (ASD). Cochrane Database Syst Rev 2016;2016(6):CD009043.
75. Maneeton N, Maneeton B, Putthisri S, et al. Risperidone for children and adolescents with autism spectrum disorder: a systematic review. Neuropsychiatr Dis Treat 2018;14:1811–20.
76. Alfageh BH, Wang Z, Mongkhon P, et al. Safety and tolerability of antipsychotic medication in individuals with autism spectrum disorder: a systematic review and meta-analysis. Paediatr Drugs 2019;21(3):153–67.
77. Fraguas D, Díaz-Caneja CM, Pina-Camacho L, et al. Dietary interventions for autism spectrum disorder: a meta-analysis. Pediatrics 2019;144(5):e20183218.

Attention Deficit and Hyperactivity Disorder

Tina Fawns, MD

KEYWORDS

- Inattentiveness versus hyperactivity • Parent-based modification programs
- ADHD coach • Interventional training • 504 Plan • Mindfulness • Working memory
- Internalizing versus externalizing symptoms

KEY POINTS

- *Diagnostic and Statistical Manual of Mental Disorders* (Fifth Edition) criteria of 6 symptoms for 6 months in 2 or more social environments.
- Multiple comorbidities from illness, including depression, anxiety, substance abuse, conduct disorder, and oppositional defiant disorder.
- School-based programs to assist: 504 Plan versus Individualized Educational Program.
- Psychosocial interventions play an important role as well as medications.
- Parent training primary treatment until age 6, then consider medication as means of intervention.

DEFINITION OF ATTENTION-DEFICIT/HYPERACTIVE DISORDER

Attention-deficit/hyperactive disorder or ADHD is defined as a neurobehavioral or neurodevelopmental disorder that is characterized by a persistent pattern of inattention and/or hyperactivity and occurs in more than 1 setting (eg, home, school, when with friends or other social environments).[1,2]

Mean onset is at 6 to 7 years of age. Approximately one-third of affected children will carry this disorder into adulthood. ADHD has a worldwide prevalence of 5% in school-aged children, and approximately 8% in the United States. ADHD is twice as common in boys than it is in girls. There appears to be a hereditary component of approximately 76%, but the exact genotype or genetic pattern has not been located.

Attention-deficit/hyperactivity disorder is the most common behavioral conditions and the second most common chronic illness in children. It is now recognized as a life-long disorder. ADHD remains a largely clinical diagnosis. Current recommendations for diagnostic evaluation of possible ADHD include a comprehensive history taking of prenatal, perinatal, and family history; school performance; environmental

Department of Family and Community Medicine at the University of Kentucky, UK HealthCare: Turfland Medical Center, 1095 Harrodsburg Road, Lexington, KY 40502, USA
E-mail address: tdfawn@gmail.com

Prim Care Clin Office Pract 48 (2021) 475–491
https://doi.org/10.1016/j.pop.2021.05.004
0095-4543/21/© 2021 Elsevier Inc. All rights reserved.

factors; and a detailed physical examination. During the physical examination, particular attention should be paid to cardiovascular and neurologic systems. Mental health assessment to probe for comorbid conditions is crucial. Last, teacher- or parent-reported behavior rating scales have been used since the 1960s to look for defined behavioral criteria.

The objective assessments currently available for ADHD are of limited use in clarifying the diagnosis. These assessments include neuropsychological tests, electroencephalogram, or neuroimaging.

PATHOPHYSIOLOGY OF ATTENTION-DEFICIT/HYPERACTIVITY DISORDER

Extensive research has shown that there are clear differences in brain size as well as activity level in the catecholamine system.[2] Animal models, neuroimaging, and pharmacologic studies have provided support for the involvement of dopaminergic and adrenergic derangements in ADHD. Also, there are differences in the mean volumes of the prefrontal cortex, the basal ganglia, and the cerebellar vermis for groups of patients with ADHD compared with unaffected controls.

In addition, risk for ADHD is increased by environmental factors, including prematurity, maternal alcohol use, smoking during pregnancy, childhood lead exposure, history of encephalitis, and head trauma.[2]

HOW DOES WORKING MEMORY DYSFUNCTION PLAY A ROLE IN ATTENTION-DEFICIT/HYPERACTIVITY DISORDER

A collaborative study performed in 2018 among 3 universities showed that organizational problems are a critical yet understudied area of impairment for children with ADHD.[3] Children with ADHD frequently show organization impairments related to planning tasks, tracking assignments, recalling due dates, and managing supplies. As a result, these children frequently misplace materials, come to class unprepared, and have messy and disorganized lockers, backpacks, and desks. In fact, the *Diagnostic and Statistical Manual of Mental Disorders* (Fifth Edition) criteria relate several symptoms that are related to disorganization. Interestingly, children with the disorder do not report organizational difficulties, but objective observers are consistent in doing so.

Working memory refers to active manipulation of information held in short-term memory. It requires the interrelated functions of the midlateral prefrontal cortex that guide behavior via the updating, processing, and temporal/sequential manipulation of internally held information. Relevant to pediatric ADHD, working memory serves as the interface between the environment and long-term memory. Working memory underlies a myriad of learning skills, including note taking, listening comprehension, and following directions. Working memory abilities also support behavioral outcomes affected by ADHD, including impulse control, cooperating with others, dynamic social decoding, and delayed tolerance. Experimental studies suggest a potential causal role of working memory dysfunction for evoking ADHD-related inattentive and hyperactive behavior.

In other words, organizational and social problems in ADHD may not reflect a lack of knowledge, but rather difficulty implementing their knowledge in the moment. Using behavioral techniques that circumvent working memory assists patients with ADHD. These organizational interventions include making written lists, breaking down multi-step instructions, providing explicit reminders, and using redirection (**Table 1**).

The *Diagnostic and Statistical Manual of Mental Disorders* requires *6 or more symptoms for at least 6 months and in more than one social setting*.[1] For adolescents,

Table 1	
Diagnostic criteria for attention-deficit/hyperactivity disorder	
Inattentiveness	**Hyperactivity/Impulsivity**
Difficulty paying attention to details	Fidgets/squirms
Making careless mistakes	Has trouble staying seated
Short attention span	Excessive running, climbing, or restlessness
Difficulty with listening	Trouble with quiet activities
Often unable to follow-through on tasks	Needs to be on the go
Avoid tasks requiring sustained mental effort	Talks too much
Often loses things	Blurts out answers
Easily distracted	Difficulty awaiting turn
Difficulty planning ahead	Interrupts conversations/intrudes on others
Appearing not to listen to caregiver or teacher	Impulsivity, including not thinking through decisions or long-term consequences. For example, engaging in sexual activities without considering the risks in adolescence
Difficulty with time management and meeting deadlines	Seeking out highly rewarding activities and peer approval leading to risky actions related to driving and substance abuse. Having a heightened response to reward and underdeveloped cognitive control in adolescence
Overscheduled	Emotional lability/lose temper easily
Forgetful in completing regular duties	Quits jobs or ends relationships prematurely
Poor organization in the home or at work	Is excessively loud or makes excessive noise during leisurely activities
Poor follow-through with task completion	Engaged in frequent or intense physical activity

Data from Refs.[1,4,5]

symptoms must have been present before 12 years of age. According to the *Diagnostic and Statistical Manual of Mental Disorders* (Fourth Edition), individuals 17 and older can be diagnosed with 5 symptoms instead of 6, with other criteria the same.

Neuropsychological testing does not increase diagnostic accuracy. However, combining direct clinical observation and parent interviews, along with parent and teacher rating scales increases diagnostic accuracy. Most common rating scores are the Conner and Vanderbilt rating scales.

COMORBID CONDITIONS ASSOCIATED WITH ATTENTION-DEFICIT/HYPERACTIVITY DISORDER

- Depression
- Anxiety
- Substance abuse
- Oppositional defiant disorder (ODD) or conduct disorder (CD)
- Poor self-esteem

- Increased injuries and accidents

If comorbid conditions are not identified and addressed, they may complicate the patient's level of functional impairment and lead to higher morbidity with poor prognosis.[6] The Childhood Behavior Checklist is a possible screening tool to look for other underlying comorbidities.

Depression

Overall, children with ADHD were 5 times more likely to have depression.[7,8] Many of the inattentive symptoms of ADHD, which include low energy, low self-esteem, difficulty concentrating, social withdrawal, tearfulness, and increased desire for sleep, can be manifestations of depression. An observer may see classic ADHD signs of disorganization and carelessness and construe them as a reflection of feeling unmotivated because of a major depression. Tearfulness could be construed as a sign of deep hopelessness rather than an intense and extreme emotional response. Most importantly, girls with ADHD react to the isolation by internalizing their disappointment rather than talking about it or acting out. Internalizing these feelings often results in feelings of despair and demoralization. It reflects the pain of being long misunderstood. Depressive features may well require treatment, but it should be treated within the context of underlying ADHD.

Anxiety

Overall, children with ADHD are 3 times more likely to have anxiety. Individuals with this diagnosis may be worried about school. Often, it is in middle school that ADHD high IQ achievers begin to falter.[7,8] Underachievement becomes a self-perpetuating entity that often continues throughout adolescence and undermines self-esteem. A more complex curriculum, multiple teachers, less overt nurturance, and multiple classrooms all require more self-direction, greater organization, efficient memory, appropriate prioritizing, and quicker transitions. All of these are challenges with individuals with ADHD. In addition, social interactions increase in complexity. There is a significant decrease in the amount of externally imposed structural guidance and a need for greater self-regulation and independence. Given the differences in executive brain function affecting these individuals, the following tasks are impacted: ability to complete multistep assignments, planning ahead, anticipating consequences, prioritizing, working independently, sustaining effort and motivation, recalling and retrieving information, transitioning from 1 subject to another, managing time, and staying organized. These school demands increase in complexity during the transition to middle school and high school. Therefore, regardless of the innate intelligence of the individual with ADHD, they will need more practice and effort to regulate these executive functions.

Rapid speech, irritability, motor restlessness, avoidant behavior, ruminating or obsessing, exaggerated fears, difficulty sleeping, and episodes of panic can all be presentations of both anxiety and ADHD. Anxiety is also a reasonable response to the relentless job of trying to compensate for ADHD difficulties. Therefore, anxiety may be an appropriate response to facing the overall increased demands of trying to keep up in school. It is possible that the secondary anxiety may resolve itself as the ADHD is treated. However, some may have 2 separate conditions, and each will need to be addressed individually, in the context of each other.

Substance Abuse

Most of the children and adolescents with ADHD who died by suicide had comorbid substance use disorder and other psychiatric diagnoses.[6,8,9] In adulthood, marijuana use and daily smoking were more prevalent in ADHD patients. The cumulative record revealed more early substance abuse of alcohol, cigarettes, marijuana, and illicit drugs in this population. Alcohol and illicit drug use escalated faster in ADHD patients in early adolescence. Early substance abuse screening and prevention in this group are critical.

The desire to be accepted by peers is particularly intense for ADHD students and adolescents. They perceive themselves as different from their peers, and therefore, are even more determined to achieve a sense of belonging. Fueled by this motivation, they are willing to go to great lengths to make themselves attractive to others. They may find themselves drawn to cigarettes, alcohol, and other drugs for peer acceptance. Alarmingly, for some, these patterns began as early as age 11. Addictive behaviors satisfy impulses, while at the same time providing high stimulation. Repetitive and impulsive behaviors serve as a way of creating order and structure out of chaos. Substance use may also relax individuals with ADHD who already feel anxious about their interpersonal skills.

Oppositional Defiant Disorder or Conduct Disorder

ADHD children are 10 times more likely to have ODD or CD. ODD/CD is associated with criminal activity and risky sexual behavior.[7] This condition is reflective of hyperactive symptoms of ADHD. Impulsivity, need for instant gratification, and need for intense physical activity owing to restlessness contribute to possible ODD/CD. These individuals have difficulty complying with social norms.

GENDER DIFFERENCES IN ATTENTION-DEFICIT/HYPERACTIVITY DISORDER

Although ADHD is 2 to 3 times more prevalent in boys than girls, a greater understanding of the clinical presentation of ADHD in girls is needed.[7] There is a higher rate of comorbid anxiety disorders and relatively lower CDs in girls compared with boys. Furthermore, relative to girls, boys with ADHD are more likely to be referred for treatment, reflecting a general delay in recognizing, diagnosing, and treating ADHD in girls that contributes to more severe symptoms among referred girls. Overall, girls have higher rates of internalizing versus externalizing disorders. In girls, treatment of internalizing symptoms is prioritized even when externalizing symptoms are present. However, externalizing symptoms are more impairing and produce worse outcomes, such as risky sexual behavior or substance abuse. It is important not to undermine timely detection and treatment of both internalizing and externalizing symptoms. Internalizing symptoms leads to development of anxiety and depression, whereas externalizing symptoms refer to acting out, such as in ODD or CD.

CRITERIA FOR STARTING ANY FORM OF MEDICATION FOR ATTENTION-DEFICIT/HYPERACTIVITY DISORDER

1. When the child's attentional difficulties are so great that he or she is unable to learn and keep up academically.[10,11]
2. When ADHD causes severe social difficulties. Sometimes ADHD children's difficulty in paying attention to social signals and impulsiveness causes significant problems with making and keeping friends.
3. When behavior at home has a seriously disruptive effect on family life, causing significant problems for the child, parents, and/or siblings.
4. When a child's self-esteem is suffering to a significant degree because of this condition.

Developed by Sandy Newmark, MD, a Clinical Professor in the Department of Pediatrics at the University of California and Director of Clinical Services at the Osher Center for Integrative Medicine.

THE DECISION TO TREAT ATTENTION-DEFICIT/HYPERACTIVITY DISORDER WITH STIMULANT MEDICATION

The decision to treat ADHD with stimulant medication should be made with the parents after a discussion of the expected benefits and potential risks. Factors such as the child's age, severity of symptoms, and comorbidities should be considered and may influence the choice of medications.[6]

Cardiac Implications of Stimulant Use for Attention-Deficit/Hyperactivity Disorder

The use of stimulants should be avoided in patients with known structural cardiac abnormalities, cardiomyopathy, serious heart rhythm abnormalities, coronary artery disease, or other serious cardiac problems that could put them at increased risk of sympathomimetic effects.[12–14] Findings from the history or physical examination that suggest cardiac disease may warrant evaluation by a cardiologist first. The American Academy of Pediatrics recommends against performing routine electrocardiogram (EKG) or routine cardiology referrals before initiating stimulant therapy, except when a workup is warranted by the examination and history.

The personal history should include questions about the following: history of fainting or dizziness, high blood pressure, heart murmur, congenital or other heart problems, seizure history, rheumatic fever, chest pain or shortness of breath with exercise, decrease in exercise tolerance, palpitations or fast heart rate, skipped beats, viral illness associated with chest pain or palpitations, current medication, and supplement use.

Family history should include questions about sudden or unexplained death in a young person; sudden cardiac death, heart attacks, or event requiring resuscitation in persons younger than aged 35 years, death during exercise, hypertrophic or other cardiomyopathy, long or short QT syndromes, or Brugada syndrome; Wolfe Parkinson-White syndrome, or other abnormal rhythm conditions; and Marfan syndrome.

The physical examination should include evaluation for the presence of an abnormal heart murmur, cardiovascular abnormalities, and Marfan syndrome. Because some cardiac conditions may not be detectable on routine physical examination, EKG may be useful because it can increase the probability of identifying children with a cardiac condition. If possible, the EKG should be read by a physician with expertise in reading EKGs in children. Before initiating therapy with a stimulant, an evaluation by a cardiologist should be done if there are any significant findings on physical examination, EKG, or patient or family history.

A recent guideline from the American Heart Association recommended routine EKG in children before they begin stimulant pharmacotherapy for ADHD. That recommendation contradicts the evidence-based recommendations from the American Academy of Child and Adolescent Psychiatry and the American Academy of Pediatrics. These organizations concluded that cardiac death in persons taking medications for ADHD is rare, with rates no higher than those in the general population of children and adolescents.

There is no evidence that routine EKG screening before beginning medical therapy for ADHD prevents sudden death.[13] Furthermore, limiting children's access to effective ADHD treatment could have serious implications (eg, substance abuse, academic problems).

Furthermore, there has been no established association between sudden cardiac death and medicines to treat ADHD.[13] Of Of 2.5 million children and adolescents of whom took stimulants for ADHD over 5 years, 19 died suddenly. These deaths resulted in a base rate of fewer than 2 incidents per year per 1 million children. Reported sudden cardiac death rates in the general child and adolescent population are substantially higher (**Table 2**).

FOOD AND DRUG ADMINISTRATION–APPROVED MEDICATIONS FOR THE TREATMENT OF ATTENTION-DEFICIT/HYPERACTIVITY DISORDER IN CHILDREN AND ADOLESCENTS

Adverse Reactions Common to all Stimulant Medications

- Decreased appetite[6]
- Insomnia
- Increased heart rate
- Headache

Stimulants

Immediate Release Stimulants	Sustained-Release and Long-Acting Stimulants
Dexmethylphenidate (Focalin)	Amphetamine/dextroamphetamine salts (Adderall)
Dextroamphetamine (Dexedrine)	Adderall XR
Methylphenidate (Ritalin)	Dexmethylphenidate (Focalin XR)
	Dextroamphetamine (Dexedrine XR)
	Lisdexamfetamine (Vyvanse)
	Methylphenidate (Concerta and Daytrana patch)
	Metadate CD
	Metadate ER
	Methylin ER
	Ritalin LA

FOOD AND DRUG ADMINISTRATION–APPROVED NONSTIMULANTS FOR THE TREATMENT OF ATTENTION-DEFICIT/HYPERACTIVITY DISORDER

- Atomoxetine (Strattera)[6]

    Side effects: Nausea, vomiting, gastrointestinal pain, anorexia, dizziness, somnolence, skin rash, pruritus, increased heart rate or blood pressure, urinary retention, or severe liver injury (rare)

    Dosing:

    [6 years old and older, less than 70 kg]

    Dose: 1.2 mg/kg/d orally divided once or twice a day; start: 0.5 mg/kg per dose orally every morning for at least 3 days; maximum: 1.4 mg/kg/d; information: in CYP2D6 poor metabolizers, start 0.5 mg/kg/dose orally every morning for 4 weeks; do not open cap; periodically reassess need for treatment

    [6 years old and older, greater than 70 kg]

    Dose: 80 mg/d orally divided once or twice a day; start: 40 mg orally every morning for at least 3 days; maximum: 100 mg/d; information: may increase to 100 mg/d after 2 to 4 weeks; in CYP2D6 poor metabolizers, start 40 mg orally every morning for 4 weeks; do not open cap; periodically reassess need for treatment[15]

Table 2
Stimulant dosing chart

Immediate Release Stimulants	Starting Dose	Titration and Timing of Doses (Always Titrate to Minimal Effective Dose)
Adderall	Children 3–5 y of age: 2.5 mg per day Age 6 y and over: 5 mg per day or twice daily	Titrate not greater than 2.5 mg/per day dose per week. Maximum dose: 40 mg Titrate no greater than 5 mg/per day dose per week. Maximum: 40 mg
Focalin *Dexmethylphenidate*	Age 6 and above: 2.5 mg twice per day	Increase weekly in increments of 2.5 mg to 5 mg per day. Maximum dose: 20 mg per day
Dexedrine *Dextroamphetamine*	Children 3–5 y of age: 2.5 mg per day Children 6–12 y of age: 5 mg once daily Adolescents and adults: 5 mg once or twice daily	Increase weekly in increments of 2.5 mg per day. Maximum dose: 20 mg Weekly increments of 5 mg per day. Maximum dose: 40 mg
Ritalin *Methylphenidate*	Children 6–12 y of age: 5 mg twice daily Adolescents the same	Increase weekly by 5 mg to 10 mg per day Maximum dose: 60 mg

Sustained-Release and Long-Acting Stimulants	Starting Dose	Titration and Timing of Doses (Always Titrate to Minimal Effective Dose)
Ritalin LA	For ages 6 and over: 10–20 mg	Increase in weekly increments by no more than 10 mg per day. Maximum dose: 60 mg
Adderall XR *Amphetamine-Dextroamphetamine Salt*	Children 6–12 y: 10 mg Above 12 y: 20 mg	For ages 6 y and above: Dose may be increased weekly by 5–10 mg per day Maximum dose: 30 mg
Focalin XR *Dexmethylphenidate*	Children 6–12 y Adolescents: 5 mg per day	Increase weekly in increments of 5 mg day Maximum dosage of 30 mg per day
Dexedrine XR Dextroamphetamine		Add 5 mg of extended-release or immediate-release formulation to the morning dose Maximum dose: 40 mg per day
Concerta Methylphenidate	Children 6–12 y and adolescents: 18 mg per day	Increase in weekly increments of 18 mg day Maximum dose: 54 mg in children 6–12 y and 72 mg in adolescents
Quillivant Methylphenidate	Children 6 y and over: 20-mg dose	Increase in weekly increments of 10–20 mg day Maximum dose: 60 mg
Vyvanse Lisdexamfetamine	Children 6 y and older: 30 mg in morning	Increase weekly in increments of 10–20 mg per day Maximum dose: 70 mg daily

Data from Sharma A, Couture J. A review of the pathophysiology, etiology, and treatment of attention-deficit hyperactivity disorder (ADHD). Ann Pharmacother. 2014 Feb;48(2):209-25.

- Guanfacine Extended Release (Intuniv)
  Side Effects: Somnolence in up to 38% of patients, headache, fatigue, upper
  abdominal pain, nausea, lethargy, dizziness, irritability, decreased blood
  pressure, decreased appetite
  Dosing: 1 mg once per day and increase by up to 1 mg per week to a maximum
  of 4 mg

ALTERNATIVE MEDICATIONS FOR THE TREATMENT OF ATTENTION-DEFICIT/ HYPERACTIVITY DISORDER IN CHILDREN AND ADOLESCENTS
Bupropion

Side effects: Sedation, constipation, dry mouth, may lower seizure threshold.[6]

- Bupropion Regular Formulation (Wellbutrin)
  Dosing: 1.4 to 2 mg per kg per day, usually 37.5 or 50 mg twice per day. Grad-
  ually increase over 2 weeks to 6 mg/kg per day up to 250 mg per day in
  divided doses. Adolescents may increase up to 300 to 400 mg per day
- Bupropion Sustained Released Formulation (Wellbutrin SR)
- Bupropion Extended-Release Formulation (Wellbutrin XL)
  Dosing of sustained released forms: 3 mg/kg per day up to 150 mg per day.
  Adolescents may increase over 2 weeks to 450 mg per day

Clonidine (Catapres)
  Side effects: Sedation, rashes with skin patch, orthostatic hypotension and less
  than 5%
  Dosing: 0.05 mg per day. Increase weekly in increments of 0.05 per day up to
  0.3 mg/d

Desipramine (Norpramin) and *Imipramine* (Tofranil)
  Side effects: Cardiac conduction disturbances, dry mouth, urinary retention,
  headache
  Dosing: 0.5–1 mg/kg per day in divided doses. Increase weekly in increments of
  1 mg/kg up to 4 mg per day divided doses preferred

Guanfacine (Tenex)
  Side effects: Fatigue, headache, insomnia
  Dosing: 0.5 to 1 mg per day. Increase by 0.5 mg every 3 to 4 days, to a maximum
  of 4 mg per day in divided doses

Psychosocial Treatments for Attention-Deficit/Hyperactivity Disorder
- Parent training[6,16]
- Individualized training interventions
- Social skills training clinics
- Alternative modalities

Parent training
Parent training behavioral modification is strongly recommended in the parents of preschool to middle school children with behavioral concerns, including ADHD. Parent
training behavioral modification addresses appropriate clear expectations and limits,
strengthens the parent-child relationship, and supports behavior change via positive
reinforcement and extinctions techniques. There must be consistent routines and
discipline across caregivers. Focus must be given to positive behaviors and ignoring
of minor negative behaviors. There must be consequences for targeted negative behaviors, confidence building, and support of successful behavior. The primary

treatment of ADHD in preschool children consists of consequences for targeted negative behaviors, building confidence, and support of successful behavior.

Training interventions

Training interventions focus on improving organization, time management, and interpersonal skills and work best for middle school or high school children. These interventions include homework coaching, practicing skills in a monitored environment, and in-depth longitudinal interventions. An ADHD coach can help patients get past obstacles and reach their goals.

Social skills training

Children with ADHD may benefit from social skills training in clinics, schools, summer camps, or an individual counseling setting. This training focuses on initiating, building, and maintaining successful relationships with peers. Methods include role play, modeling, practice, and positive feedback. Social skills groups seem to be most effective when used with other intervention programs, either parenting or school based.

The focus of social skills would be to learn how to listen without interrupting, showing the patient the importance of listening and letting others finish what they are saying, the importance of eye contact and focusing on what is being said, and respecting others' space and keeping their volume at an acceptable level so as to not interfere with others' conversations.

Alternative Modalities

Alternative therapies focus on mindfulness, cognitive behavior therapy, diet, herbal supplements, behavioral modifications, biofeedback, and supportive counseling (Table 3).[6,10,11] In addition, neurofeedback, a form of biofeedback, uses electroencephalograph biofeedback to teach children how to self-regulate certain brain activity patterns and then generalize these skills to daily life.

Mindfulness

There has been a great deal of recent interest and use of modalities like *meditation*, *yoga*, and *aia chi* for the treatment of ADHD.[11] Several small studies have shown positive results especially with mindfulness meditation. Although systemic results have noted a lack of randomized trials, it is considered an important area future research.[17]

A study by Kuo and Taylor[14] in 2004 evaluated the lack of *nature and green space* as partially responsible for the increase of ADHD and other mental disorders. It surveyed

Table 3 Modalities			
Mindfulness	Herbals/ Botanicals	Supplements	Diet
Meditation	Gingko biloba	Omega-3 up to 2 g daily	Avoidance of additives and artificial flavors
Yoga	Pycnogenol	Magnesium	Low gluten diet
Thai chi	Valerian and lemon-balm for restful sleep	Zinc	Diet low in concentrated sugars
Regular exercise		Iron	Elimination diets
Natural setting or green space		Melatonin to assist with sleep	

450 parents concerning the effects of green or nongreen activities on the behavior of their children with ADHD. There was a significant tendency for the green activities to result in decreased ADHD symptoms; although the study clearly had it is limitations, it suggests a possible role for nature or natural settings having a calming effect on these patients.[18]

In 2018, a systemic review[19] of *exercise* and ADHD concluded benefits of a variety of exercise programs in improving motor skills, physical fitness, attention, and social behavior of patients with ADHD. In a study authored by Chang and colleagues[20] in 2012, children with ADHD exercised intensely for 30 minutes and then underwent a formal test of executive function. Those in the exercise group demonstrated significant improvements compared with the control group. Last, a group of ADHD children participated in physical activity training for 45 minutes 3 times a week for 10 weeks. Compared with the controls, participants had significant improved behavior ratings from teachers and parents, as well as more in formal tests of attention. This study was performed by Verret and colleagues[21] in 2012.

Botanicals

Ginkgo biloba
In a 2001 open-label study[22] of a combination of *Gingko biloba* and *Panax quinquefolius*, improvements in ADHD symptoms were shown after 4 weeks of treatment.[11] In 2015,[23] Gingko or placebo was given to 66 children who were taking Methylphenidate. After 6 weeks, those taking Gingko had significant improvement in ratings of attention. The evidence for Gingko effectiveness is therefore limited but found to be of value in some children.

Pycnogenol
Pycnogenol is a standard extract from French maritime pine tree. It is widely touted as an effective treatment for ADHD. The *European Journal of Pediatrics* published a study in 2006 by Trebatickà and colleagues[24] indicating a randomized placebo controlled and double-blind study where Pycnogenol was used in 61 children with ADHD. After 4 weeks of treatment, the treatment group improved significantly compared with placebo. Also, 1 month after treatment was discontinued, symptoms returned to baseline. The mechanism of action is proposed to be increased production of nitric oxide, which regulates dopamine and norepinephrine release and reuptake.

Valerian root and Lemon Balm
Valerian root and lemon balm have been shown in combination to assist with sleep and relaxation. In a study by Müller and Klement,[25] 918 children with hyperkinesis and dyssomnia were treated for 4 weeks with this combination, and 70% of children with hyperkinesis and 80% with insomnia improved significantly. There were no significant adverse effects. However, there was no control group. Also, these children did not have diagnosed ADHD.

Supplements

Omega-3 fatty acids
The most thoroughly researched supplements for the treatment of ADHD are Omega-3 fatty acids. It has been clearly established that children with ADHD have lower red blood cell levels of omega-3 than those who do not.[11,26] There have been many studies of the effect of omega-3 supplementation on the symptoms of ADHD. Most but not all of them show a significant positive effect. There are several unanswered questions about Omega-3 and ADHD. What is the right dose and the right ratio of

Eicosapentaenoic acid and Docosahexaenoic acid? How do you get kids to take them? There is not enough research to justify clinical recommendations as to dosing and ratios at this time.

Iron supplementation due to low ferritin

Several studies have shown that up to 84% of children with ADHD have low ferritin levels.[27,28] Moreover, ferritin levels are proportional to worse behavior in children with ADHD. Of note, studies do not find anemia, but simply low ferritin levels, which represent peripheral iron status. Iron is necessary for tyrosine hydroxylase, which is needed for dopamine synthesis, and iron deficiency is associated with decreased dopamine transporter gene expression, which has been correlated with ADHD. Given the research at this point, it makes sense to assess serum ferritin levels and treat those children who are deficient as part of an integrative approach to ADHD.

Zinc deficiency

Several studies have shown a tendency for ADHD children to be deficient in zinc, and some recent trials have confirmed the benefit of zinc supplementation.[29] However, the overall evidence for zinc is not as robust as it is for Omega-3 or iron supplementation. A large proportion of studies were done outside of the United States and Europe and may reflect zinc conditions not applicable here. In 1 randomized trial by Bilici and colleagues[30] in 2004, zinc sulfate reduced impulsive and hyperactive but not inattentive symptoms, compared with placebo. In a study by Akhondzadeh and colleagues[31] in 2004, children received a combination of zinc and methylphenidate and performed significantly better than methylphenidate alone. In a more recent study by Arnold and colleagues[32,33] in 2011, children with ADHD were given 15 to 30 mg of zinc with or without stimulant. Zinc alone was not helpful, but for those taking stimulants, the necessary dose was reduced by 37% overall. There is suggestive but not clear evidence that zinc status is important in ADHD, particularly to patients on stimulants and in the hyperactive patients more so than the inattentive.

Magnesium deficiency

Magnesium levels in both serum and hair are lower in children with ADHD. This finding has been confirmed by 2 recent meta-analyses.[34,35] There has been a significant decline in magnesium intake over the last 70 years. Fruits and vegetables now have only a fraction of the magnesium that formerly they once had, and this is true of organic vegetables as well. Magnesium reduces stress and glutamate activity. However, there have been no randomized placebo controlled trials of magnesium supplementation and ADHD. Magnesium seems to have the most benefit in addressing hyperactivity and not inattention.

Melatonin

Sleep problems, particularly increased sleep latency, are also a common complaint in many children with ADHD. When sleep is a problem, melatonin treatment is often very effective. Many well-controlled studies[35,36] have shown that melatonin is significantly better than placebo at reducing sleep onset latency in both stimulant-treated and medication-free children with ADHD. A study by Maras and colleagues[37] in 2018 indicated that melatonin was safe and effective. In a follow-up study,[38] children reported no serious adverse effects or treatment-related comorbidities associated with melatonin after follow-up of 3.7 years. Many children respond to lower doses of 1 mg or less, and recommended starting dose is 0.5 mg and is working up, if necessary. Adequate treatment of sleep often improves a child's ADHD symptoms.

Diet

Artificial food coloring, flavors, and additives/preservatives

Bateman and colleagues[39] performed a study of 273 three-year-olds with hyperactivity.[11] After an initial washout, they were given a drink with either food coloring and sodium benzoate or placebo. There was a significant statistical increase in hyperactivity in those given the active substance. McCann and colleagues[40] published a double-blind, placebo controlled study examining the effects of artificial flavoring and additives on hyperactive behavior in 3- to 4-year-old and 8- to 9-year-old children from the general population in 2007. All children had artificial flavor additives and artificial food coloring removed from their diet for a 6-week trial and then consumed either placebo or artificial coloring and additives. There was an increased global hyperactivity in the 3- to 4-year-olds and 8- to 9-year-olds after consuming the active product. Note that these were normal individuals without any behavioral diagnosis.

Sugar

The role of sugar is an area of controversy. Although many parents of children with and without ADHD notice adverse hyperactive reactions to large amounts of sugar, research has not substantiated this connection.[41] Perhaps some children are more sensitive to sugar, whereas others are not.[6]

Elimination diets (such as removal of gluten or antigenic foods)

Researchers have also examined the role of allergy or sensitivity to common foods and ADHD. Egger and colleagues[42] placed 76 children on an oligo-antigenic or a "few foods diet" in an open-label trial, and 62 of the children improved. This study was performed in 1985. In the second double-blinded placebo controlled phase of this study, those children who reacted demonstrated significantly increased ADHD symptoms when the actual offending foods compared with placebo were given. Carter and colleagues[43] performed a similar study with 59 out of 78 children improving during open trial and a positive result in the double-blinded aspect of the trial in 1993. Interestingly, artificial colors and flavors were the most common offenders in all studies. Elimination diets typically involve removal of gluten, casein, soy, corn, egg, and peanuts as well.

SCHOOL-BASED PROGRAMS FOR ATTENTION-DEFICIT/HYPERACTIVITY DISORDER

There are 2 federal civil rights laws that protect the educational rights of children with ADHD and other disabilities: Section 504 of the Rehabilitations Act of 1973 and the Individuals with Disabilities Education Act (IDEA). These laws provide guidance for the education of all students with disabilities in public schools that receive federal funds.

- Both laws guarantee children with disabilities a free appropriate public education.
- Both recommend that children be educated in the least restrictive environment with nondiscriminatory evaluations and assessments and periodic reevaluation.
- Section 504 defines disability more broadly than IDEA. It is less burdensome to qualify and may get implemented faster.
- IDEA is best known for its main provision the IEP, Individualized Educational Program. Although an IEP can offer more comprehensive educational benefits, it can be harder to qualify for and take longer to get.

ADHD qualifies as a disability in most schools because it can impact school performance. These plans outline accommodations designed to optimize learning for children with disabilities. Such accommodations can include extended test time, reduced homework, extra study materials, and supplemental class notes. Children qualify for these support services when ADHD severity impairs their ability to learn.

Additional school-based support services, such as speech or occupational therapy, are provided through individual education plans. IEPs are written agreements between parent and school that states the child's current academic and functional performance, formal learning accommodations, and measurable annual goals for what the child is supposed to achieve. As the child gets older, he or she plays a more direct role in shaping this conversation.

CLINICS CARE POINTS

- Take time to investigate and determine the primary diagnosis as well as all comorbid conditions that may be affecting behavior. This will allow for better overall management and coordination of care.

- Get a school-based program on board early, to set up the child for success. Meet with teachers and guidance counselors to discuss what works best for the promotion of the child's learning.

- Make sure to get multiple perspectives during the evaluation period. Have multiple teachers, parents, therapists, extracurricular coaches, and leaders fill out surveys to determine diagnosis and to reassess progress.

- Continue to communicate with the patient to see how they perceive the medication is working. Also, ask the patient how their perception of themselves is altered on the medication in either a positive or a negative way. Continue to monitor emotional stability.

- Medication is not the answer for everyone. Keep open to multiple modalities and assess if medication is necessary given the patient's current performance and social interactions.

DISCLOSURE

No disclosures.

REFERENCES

1. Brahmbhatt K, Hilty DM, Hah M, et al. Diagnosis and treatment of attention deficit hyperactivity disorder during adolescence in the primary care setting: a concise review. J Adolesc Health 2018;63(1):126.
2. Wolraich ML, Chan E, Froehlich t, et al. ADHD diagnosis and treatment guidelines: a historical perspective. Pediatrics 2019;144(4):1–9.
3. Kofler MJ, Sarver DE, Harmon SL, et al. Working memory and organizational skills problems in ADHD. Child Psychol Psychiatry 2018;59(1):57–67.
4. Wetterer L. Attention-deficit/hyperactivity disorder: AAP updates guideline for diagnosis and management. Am Fam Physician 2020;102(1):58–60.
5. Information from your family doctor: ADHD in children. Am Fam Physician 2009;79(8).
6. Armstrong C. ICSI releases guideline on diagnosis and management of ADHD in children. Am Fam Physician 2011;83(6):762–8.

7. Tung I, Li JJ, Meza JI, et al. Patterns of comorbidity among girls with ADHD: a meta-analysis. Pediatrics 2016;138:1–13.
8. Nadeau KG, Littman EB, Quinn PO. Understanding girls with AD/HD. 155-161. Silver Spring, MD: Advantage Books; 1999.
9. Molina BSG, Howard AL, Swanson JM, et al. Substance use through adolescence into early adulthood after childhood-diagnosed ADHD: findings from the MTA longitudinal study. J Child Psychol Psychiatry 2018;59(6):692–702.
10. Newmark S. ADHD without drugs: a guide to the natural care of children with ADHD. Nurtured Heart Publications; 2010.
11. IMR-Faculty Learner. Integrative pediatric neurology: ADHD & autism. Treatment of approaches to ADHD. Instructor Sandy Newmark. Copyright 2020 the Arizona Board of Regents on behalf of the University of Arizona. 2019. Available at: https://residency.integrativemedicine.arizona.edu/.
12. Armstrong C. AAP responds to AHA guideline on cardiovascular monitoring before starting stimulants for ADHD. Am Fam Physician 2009;79(10):910.
13. Graham Lisa. AHA releases recommendations on cardiovascular monitoring and use of ADHD medications in children with heart disease. Am Fam Physician 2009; 79(10):905–10.
14. Kuo FE, Taylor AF. A potential natural treatment for attention-deficit/hyperactivity disorder: evidence from a national study. Am J Public Health 2004;94(9):1580–6.
15. Epocrates. Available at: https://www.epocrates.com. Copyright 2020 per Aetna-Health, All rights Reserved. Assessed December 2020.
16. Felt FT, Lumeng J. Multimodal treatment of attention-deficit/hyperactivity disorder. Am Fam Physician 2009;79(8):640–1.
17. Zhang J, Díaz Román A, Cortese S. Meditation-based therapies for attention-deficit/hyperactivity disorder in children, adolescents and adults: a systematic review and meta-analysis. Evid Based Ment Health 2018;21(3):87–94.
18. Louv R. Last child in the woods: saving our children from nature-deficit disorder. New York: Algonquin Books of Chapel Hill; 2005.
19. S J, Arumugam N, Parasher RK. Effect of physical exercises on attention, motor skill and physical fitness in children with attention deficit hyperactivity disorder: a systematic review. Atten Defic Hyperact Disord 2019;11(2):125–37.
20. Chang YK, Liu S, Yu HH, et al. Effect of acute exercise on executive function in children with attention deficit hyperactivity disorder. Arch Clin Neuropsychol 2012;27(2):225–37.
21. Verret C, Guay MC, Berthiaume C, et al. A physical activity program improves behavior and cognitive functions in children with ADHD: an exploratory study. J Atten Disord 2012;16(1):71–80.
22. Lyon MR, Cline JC, Totosy de Zepetnek J, et al. Effect of the herbal extract combination Panax quinquefolium and Ginkgo biloba on attention-deficit hyperactivity disorder: a pilot study. J Psychiatry Neurosci 2001;26(3):221–8.
23. Shakibaei F, Radmanesh M, Salari E, et al. Ginkgo biloba in the treatment of attention-deficit/hyperactivity disorder in children and adolescents. A randomized, placebo-controlled, trial. Complement Ther Clin Pract 2015;21(2):61–7.
24. Trebatická J, Kopasová S, Hradecná Z, et al. Treatment of ADHD with French maritime pine bark extract, Pycnogenol. Eur Child Adolesc Psychiatry 2006; 15(6):329–35.
25. Müller SF, Klement S. A combination of valerian and lemon balm is effective in the treatment of restlessness and dyssomnia in children. Phytomedicine 2006;13(6):383–7.

26. Colter AL, Cutler C, Meckling KA. Fatty acid status and behavioural symptoms of attention deficit hyperactivity disorder in adolescents: a case-control study. Nutr J 2008;7:8.

27. Konofal E, Lecendreux M, Deron J, et al. Effects of iron supplementation on attention deficit hyperactivity disorder in children. Pediatr Neurol 2008; 38(1):20–6.

28. Oner P, Oner O, Azik FM, et al. Ferritin and hyperactivity ratings in attention deficit hyperactivity disorder. Pediatr Int 2012;54(5):688–92.

29. Villagomez A, Ramtekkar U. Iron, magnesium, vitamin D, and zinc deficiencies in children presenting with symptoms of attention-deficit/hyperactivity disorder. Children (Basel) 2014;1(3):261–79.

30. Bilici M, Yildirim F, Kandil S, et al. Double-blind, placebo-controlled study of zinc sulfate in the treatment of attention deficit hyperactivity disorder. Prog Neuropsychopharmacol Biol Psychiatry 2004;28(1):181–90.

31. Akhondzadeh S, Mohammadi MR, Khademi M. Zinc sulfate as an adjunct to methylphenidate for the treatment of attention deficit hyperactivity disorder in children: a double blind and randomized trial [ISRCTN64132371]. BMC Psychiatry 2004;4:9.

32. Arnold LE, Disilvestro RA, Bozzolo D, et al. Zinc for attention-deficit/hyperactivity disorder: placebo-controlled double-blind pilot trial alone and combined with amphetamine. J Child Adolesc Psychopharmacol 2011;21(1):1–19.

33. Huang YH, Zeng BY, Li DJ, et al. Significantly lower serum and hair magnesium levels in children with attention deficit hyperactivity disorder than controls: a systematic review and meta-analysis. Prog Neuropsychopharmacol Biol Psychiatry 2019;90:134–41.

34. Effatpanah M, Rezaei M, Effatpanah H, et al. Magnesium status and attention deficit hyperactivity disorder (ADHD): a meta-analysis. Psychiatry Res 2019; 274:228–34.

35. Corkum P, Tannock R, Moldofsky H. Sleep disturbances in children with attention-deficit/hyperactivity disorder. J Am Acad Child Adolesc Psychiatry 1998;37(6): 637–46.

36. Sung V, Hiscock H, Sciberras E, et al. Sleep problems in children with attention-deficit/hyperactivity disorder: prevalence and the effect on the child and family. Arch Pediatr Adolesc Med 2008;162(4):336–42.

37. Maras A, Schroder CM, Malow BA, et al. Long-term efficacy and safety of pediatric prolonged-release melatonin for insomnia in children with autism spectrum disorder. J Child Adolesc Psychopharmacol 2018;28(10):699–710.

38. Hoebert M, van der Heijden KB, van Geijlswijk IM, et al. Long-term follow-up of melatonin treatment in children with ADHD and chronic sleep onset insomnia. J Pineal Res 2009;47(1):1–7.

39. Bateman B, Warner JO, Hutchinson E, et al. The effects of a double blind, placebo controlled, artificial food colourings and benzoate preservative challenge on hyperactivity in a general population sample of preschool children. Arch Dis Child 2004;89(6):506–11 [Erratum in: Arch Dis Child. 2005;90(8):875].

40. McCann D, Barrett A, Cooper A, et al. Food additives and hyperactive behaviour in 3-year-old and 8/9-year-old children in the community: a randomised, double-blinded, placebo-controlled trial. Lancet 2007;370(9598):1560–7 [Erratum in: Lancet. 2007;370(9598):1542].

41. Schnoll R, Burshteyn D, Cea-Aravena J. Nutrition in the treatment of attention-deficit hyperactivity disorder: a neglected but important aspect. Appl Psychophysiol Biofeedback 2003;28(1):63–75.

42. Egger J, Carter CM, Graham PJ, et al. Controlled trial of oligoantigenic treatment in the hyperkinetic syndrome. Lancet 1985;1(8428):540–5.

43. Carter CM, Urbanowicz M, Hemsley R, et al. Effects of a few food diet in attention deficit disorder. Arch Dis Child 1993;69(5):564–8.

Adverse Childhood Experiences

Carol Hustedde, PhD

KEYWORDS

- Childhood trauma • Adverse childhood experiences (ACEs)
- Adult health risk behaviors • ACE surveillance surveys • ACE Questionnaire

KEY POINTS

- More than 60% of adults report having a least 1 adverse childhood experience and 17% report 4 or more adverse childhood experiences.
- Adverse childhood experiences affect many individuals, regardless of socioeconomic status, race, or education level.
- Adverse childhood experiences have significant, long-term effects on mental and physical health throughout the life span.
- Adverse childhood experiences have been identified in children in the child welfare system as young as 18 months of age. Adversity early in the lifespan impacts healthy neurobiological development.
- The primary care setting is the optimal environment to identify adverse childhood experiences and implement prevention strategies.

INTRODUCTION

Adverse childhood experiences (ACEs) have become a more widely studied topic in the literature,[1] although there is a prior history of relevant research studies.[2] This work has generated important and extensive knowledge about child abuse and the probable consequences of exposures to trauma during childhood. Although the seminal research[3] on this topic was published more than 20 years ago, it did not receive consistent attention from the medical community until the past 10 years or so.[4] Nonetheless, the literature has put forth a conceptual framework, as well as a screening device to identify a positive history of traumatic experiences during childhood.[3] The literature now contains numerous reports about ACEs and the significant impact of childhood adversity on child and adult health and the quality of life.[5,6] The connections between health behaviors and lifestyles to the causes of morbidity and mortality in the United States are well-known. Acknowledgment that abuse and adversities during

Department of Family and Community Medicine, University of Kentucky College of Medicine, 2150 Harrodsburg Road, Suite 125, Lexington, KY 40504, USA
E-mail address: chustedde@uky.edu

Prim Care Clin Office Pract 48 (2021) 493–504
https://doi.org/10.1016/j.pop.2021.05.005
0095-4543/21/© 2021 Elsevier Inc. All rights reserved.

childhood lead to risk factors for adults can, in turn, distinguish ACEs as the basic causes of morbidity and mortality during adulthood.[3]

The original work that led to the current knowledge base about ACEs was inspired by a study about obesity,[7,8] conducted by Felliti at Kaiser Permanente in California. One hundred obese patients participated in interviews about how their obesity was related to life events when they applied to participate in a very low calorie program. Interview results showed that these individuals had a very high level of childhood emotional and sexual abuse, suffered from early loss of a parent, parental substance abuse, and domestic violence. These findings were important as to their applicability to the patients' medical treatment for obesity and other health issues.

Felitti was joined by the Centers for Disease Control and Prevention to expand the study on obese patients to a much broader sample of adults who received primary care services from Kaiser Permanente. This landmark study[3] surveyed about 13,500 patients (70.5% response rate) after they completed a standardized medical examination. The researchers sought to examine the relationship between 7 categories of ACEs (**Fig. 1**), to high-risk health behaviors, disease, and overall health status. The data were then analyzed to predict the relationship between the total number of abuse categories and the major causes of death for adults. The results from this analysis were definitive, because more than one-half of the participants reported at least 1 category of childhood exposures and one-quarter of the participants reported 2 or more categories.

There was a significant relationship between the number of categories of childhood exposure and each of the adult health risk behaviors. In addition, the presence of 1 significantly increased the prevalence of having additional ACEs.[9] Felitti[3] selected 10 risk behaviors for analysis owing to their roles in rates of adult morbidity and mortality in the United States,[10] and they included smoking, depression, alcoholism, and a high number of sexual partners, as well as 6 additional high-risk behaviors. Felitti first described a dose–response relationship that existed between the number of identified ACEs and high-risk health behaviors, so that greater exposure to ACEs was correlated with greater health risks.[3,9] When study participants who

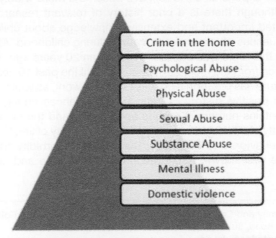

Fig. 1. Categories of ACEs. (*Adapted from* Felitti VJ, Anda RF, Nordenberg D, Williamson DF, Spitz AM, Edwards V, Koss MP, Marks JS. Relationship of childhood abuse and household dysfunction to many of the leading causes of death in adults. The Adverse Childhood Experiences (ACE) Study. Am J Prev Med. 1998 May;14(4):245-58; with permission.)

had 4 or more categories of childhood exposures were compared with participants with no exposures, their risks for alcoholism, drug abuse, depression, and attempted suicide increased between 4- and 12-fold. **Fig. 2** depicts the harmful impact of ACEs from childhood to adulthood.

The Centers for Disease Control and Prevention–Kaiser Permanente study established the topic of ACEs in the research world, and, in the past 20 years or so, many researchers have contributed to a large body of literature that attempts to better understand how this issue impacts clinical care, public health and public policy. Hughes and colleagues[11] and Zarse and colleagues[12] published comprehensive reviews of the literature to identify adult health outcomes as measured by the ACE questionnaire developed by Felitti and colleagues. Because the knowledge base has grown dramatically, the literature has begun to also put forth challenges about the usefulness of ACEs conceptually and for screening applications.[2,13,14]

SCREENING FOR ADVERSE CHILDHOOD EXPERIENCES
Adults

The first screening device was developed by Felitti and colleagues[3] as a part of their large study with Kaiser Permanente patients. Referred to as The ACEs Study Questionnaire, it has 17 individual questions (**Box 1**) that are grouped according to adversity type. It is a retrospective assessment of adult patients about their experiences with different forms of abuse when they were between the ages 0 to 17 years. The scoring is simple: each positive response accounts for 1 ACE. The ACEs Study Questionnaire, as well as modifications made by other investigators, remains the fundamental prototype for instruments intended to screen adults, and it is often administered in a clinical or related human service setting.

At the national level, the Behavioral Risk Factor Surveillance System (BRFSS) is administered annually and is the vehicle used to survey adults about ACEs. Eleven questions about ACEs were added to the standard set of BRFSS questions.[15] The literature includes reports about the BRFSS ACE findings for different time periods and different groups of states reporting.[16] It is important to note that states differ in the frequency of collecting BRFSS ACE data.[16]

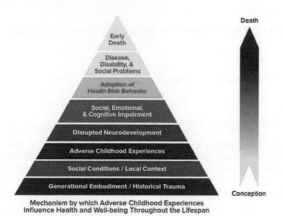

Fig. 2. The ACE pyramid. (*From* Centers for Disease Control and Prevention (CDC). Adverse Childhood Experiences Resources. Available at https://www.cdc.gov/violenceprevention/aces/resources.html. Accessed May 4, 2021.)

Box 1
ACE Questionnaire

Before your 18th birthday:

1. Did a parent or other adult in the household often or very often… Swear at you, insult you, put you down, or humiliate you? or act in a way that made you afraid that you might be physically hurt?
No___
If Yes, enter 1 __

2. Did a parent or other adult in the household often or very often… Push, grab, slap, or throw something at you? or Ever hit you so hard that you had marks or were injured?
No___
If Yes, enter 1 __

3. Did an adult or person at least 5 years older than you ever… Touch or fondle you or have you touch their body in a sexual way? or Attempt or actually have oral, anal, or vaginal intercourse with you?
No___
If Yes, enter 1 __

4. Did you often or very often feel that … No one in your family loved you or thought you were important or special? or Your family didn't look out for each other, feel close to each other, or support each other?
No___
If Yes, enter 1 __

5. Did you often or very often feel that … You didn't have enough to eat, had to wear dirty clothes, and had no one to protect you? or Your parents were too drunk or high to take care of you or take you to the doctor if you needed it?
No___
If Yes, enter 1 __

6. Were your parents ever separated or divorced?
No___
If Yes, enter 1 __

7. Was your mother or stepmother: Often or very often pushed, grabbed, slapped, or had something thrown at her? or Sometimes, often, or very often kicked, bitten, hit with a fist, or hit with something hard? or Ever repeatedly hit over at least a few minutes or threatened with a gun or knife?
No___
If Yes, enter 1 __

8. Did you live with anyone who was a problem drinker or alcoholic, or who used street drugs?
No___
If Yes, enter 1 __

9. Was a household member depressed or mentally ill, or did a household member attempt suicide?
No___
If Yes, enter 1 __

10. Did a household member go to prison?
No___
If Yes, enter 1 __

Now add up your "Yes" answers: _ This is your ACE Score_____

From Felitti VJ, Anda R, Nordenberg D, Williamson D, Spitz A, Edwards V, Koss M, Marks J. Relationship of childhood abuse and household dysfunction to many of the leading causes of death in adults: The adverse childhood experiences (ACE) Study. *Amer J Prev Med.* 1998;14(4):245-258; with permission.

Children

Historically, the assessment of ACEs has focused on retrospective responses from adults, often in mid-life, to identify their childhood exposure to ACEs. There has been significant interest in assessing ACEs in children during their childhood to measure trauma and chronic and toxic stress.[17] Such measurements can lead to important initiatives and policies to prevent ACEs and decrease the harmful effects of traumatic occurrences during childhood. The National Survey of Children's Health (NSCH) is funded and managed by the Maternal and Child Health Bureau of the Health Resources and Services Administration. It gathers national and state level estimates of key measures of child health and well-being for children ages 0 to 17 years on an annual basis.

The NSCH focused on 9 categories of ACEs[5] (**Box 2**) and added questions that ask the respondent if the child has ever experienced one or more ACEs, and the findings were first reported for the 2016 NSHC survey.[18] The NSCH is administered as a household survey by asking a parent or guardian who is familiar with the child to identify the presence of ACEs in the home.

PREVALENCE OF ADVERSE CHILDHOOD EXPERIENCES

Adults

Much of what is known about the prevalence of ACEs for adults comes from the BRFSS. Merrick and colleagues[19] reported on data collected from 23 states that gathered responses to 11 ACEs questions. Approximately 214,000 adults participated and 61.55% had a least 1 ACE and 26.64% reported 3 or more ACEs. For participants who identified as Black, Hispanic, or multiracial, the number of ACEs was significantly higher. This finding also held true for adults who had less than a high school education, those with low incomes, and those who were unemployed or unable to work. Individuals who identified as a sexual minority had much higher exposures to ACEs than did those who identified as white, who were employed and identified as straight.

Box 2
Categories of ACEs as measured by the NSCH

Somewhat often/very often hard to get by on income

Parent/guardian divorced or separated

Parent/guardian died

Parent/guardian served time in jail

Saw or heard violence in the home

Victim of violence or witnessed neighborhood violence

Lived with anyone mentally ill, suicidal, or depressed

Lived with anyone with alcohol or drug problem

Often treated unfairly owing to race/ethnicity

From Bethell, CD, Davis, MB, Gombojav, N, Stumbo, S, Powers, K. Issue Brief: A national and across state profile on adverse childhood experiences among children and possibilities to heal and thrive. Baltimore: Johns Hopkins Bloomberg School of Public Health, 2017; with permission.

Some investigators have questioned whether prior research about the prevalence of ACEs can be generalized to the increasingly diverse populations in the United States.[20] Because individuals of Hispanic descent now make up the nation's largest ethnic or racial minority group,[21] it is important to understand the trauma and adversity that Latinos have experienced. LaBrenz and colleagues[20] suggested that family composition and the role of family could impact the link between ACEs and health outcomes as well as competence as parents or caregivers. This study reported that the ACE scores for this population are related to mental health issues and substance use, and that individuals with an ACE score of 4 or 5 had lower levels of parenting competence than those with an ACE score of zero.

Children

Many reports have documented the prevalence of ACEs in the United States. On a national level, data show that 34 million children, or 50% of all children between the ages of 0 and 17, faced at least 1 ACE.[5] More than 20% suffered from 2 or more ACEs.[5] ACEs are identified in children who are insured by either public or private insurers; however, the prevalence is much higher for children who receive public health insurance. Children at all points of the socioeconomic continuum are identified with ACEs, and, not surprisingly, the percentage is higher for children who live in impoverished homes. Using data from the 2016 NSCH indicated that the most prevalent forms of ACEs for a sample of more than 45,000 children were economic hardship and parent or guardian divorce or separation. In addition, 5 sample characteristics were shown to impact outcomes for all children: the child's age, poverty, family makeup, type of health insurance, and presence of special health care needs.[18]

Rural children have higher rates of exposure to ACEs than do children who live in urban settings,[22] and the majority of these children were non-Hispanic White and less likely to be non-Hispanic African American. Urban children were found to live with a single mother more frequently than rural children, whereas a greater number of rural children had a parent with a high school education or less.

Data about children in the child welfare system are especially troubling. It has been reported that children between the ages of 18 and 71 months had, on average, 3.6 ACEs and were linked to poor mental health and chronic medical issues.[23] Children between the ages of 36 and 71 months were identified to be at greater risk for impaired social development. This finding supports the usefulness of screening for ACEs in children rather than sole reliance on retrospective reports from adults.

Childhood, as a time period, is very vulnerable, and evidence of abuse and adversity appears in both the biological[24,25] and behavioral systems of children.[26] When children are exposed to adversities without protection, the timing, intensity, and cumulative burden of ACEs can affect gene expression, the conditioning of stress responses, and the development of immune system function.[27] Repeated stress in children as a result of adversity can bring about high levels of stress hormones, such as cortisol or norepinephrine, which can be protective; however, when they are released for longer durations, they become toxic. The wear and tear on organ systems and other recovery processes can lead to allostatic load.[28,29]

ADULT MORBIDITIES ASSOCIATED WITH ADVERSE CHILDHOOD EXPERIENCES

The relationship between ACEs and high-risk behaviors of adults revealed that adults with an ACE score greater than 4 had a greater risk for heavy or binge drinking, smoking, risky HIV behavior, myocardial infarction, stroke, depression, coronary heart disease, diabetes, disability owing to a health condition, and the need for special equipment to manage the disability.[30] ACE scores are also linked to not only lower cessation rates in people with serious health problems owing to smoking, but also a greater risk of having more smoking-induced medical diseases.[31]

Much of what is known about the connection between ACEs and poor health status in adults has been collected from population samples that were predominately White and were, on average, around 57 years old.[32] ACE scores from a group of just more than 1000 urban, minority young adults between the ages of 22 and 24 were determined based on a dataset composed of longitudinal data (Chicago Longitudinal Study) that described the development of racial and ethnic minority children in low-income, urban families.[33] Approximately 80% of the participants experienced at least 1 ACE, and 50% were exposed to multiple ACEs. The evidence showed that increased exposure to ACEs was linked to a greater probability of poor overall health and mental health, along with substance use in young, minority adults.

Prevention

More recently, published studies have begun to describe strategies to prevent or decrease the occurrence of ACEs in children.[15,34] The Centers for Disease Control and Prevention developed a comprehensive public health methodology using 6 strategies to prevent ACEs based on the best evidence available.[35] **Fig. 3** lists the strategies.

Preventing ACEs

Strategy	Approach
Strengthen economic supports to families	• Strengthening household financial security • Family-friendly work policies
Promote social norms that protect against violence and adversity	• Public education campaigns • Legislative approaches to reduce corporal punishment • Bystander approaches • Men and boys as allies in prevention
Ensure a strong start for children	• Early childhood home visitation • High-quality child care • Preschool enrichment with family engagement
Teach skills	• Social-emotional learning • Safe dating and healthy relationship skill programs • Parenting skills and family relationship approaches
Connect youth to caring adults and activities	• Mentoring programs • After-school programs
Intervene to lessen immediate and long-term harms	• Enhanced primary care • Victim-centered services • Treatment to lessen the harms of ACEs • Treatment to prevent problem behavior and future involvement in violence • Family-centered treatment for substance use disorders

Fig. 3. Evidence-based prevention and mitigation strategies for ACEs. (*From* Centers for Disease Control and Prevention (CDC). Preventing Adverse Childhood Experiences: Leveraging the Best Available Evidence. Atlanta, GA: National Center for Injury Prevention and Control, Centers for Disease Control and Prevention. 2019.)

Resilience, or the ability to remain calm when dealing with adversity, may serve to lessen the impact of ACEs during childhood.[1] Bethell and colleagues[1] measured the connections between ACEs and childhood chronic conditions, health risks, and success in school. In addition, they evaluated the potential effects of resilience on these children when they are able to access medical care in a family-centered medical home. Children with ACEs were less likely to demonstrate resilience than children without ACEs and were less likely to have a protective home environment with healthy parents who were not always annoyed with them. When children with ACEs did not receive health care in a family-centered medical home, they also were less likely to show evidence of resilience.

A systematic review of randomized controlled trials indicated that many models of prevention include parenting education, referrals to social services, and social support for families with children ages 0 to 5 years.[36] Of importance is the premise that the effect of ACEs on health outcomes is mediated by how much ACEs influence the parent–child relationship. Therefore, interventions that improve the parent–child relationship are key to preventing or decreasing the impact of ACEs. Another important conclusion is that, because ACEs affect individuals at all points on the socioeconomic continuum, interventions will need to be appropriate for individuals at various income levels.

Health care providers have a role in the prevention or reduction of harm caused by ACEs[37,38] and should pursue training about ACEs to become familiar with prevention strategies and how to care for patients who have ACEs. Many clinicians do not screen for ACEs because they have not become confident about the screening process and hesitate to talk to patients about ACEs. Health care settings often lack the resources that would provide support for victims of ACEs, and clinicians worry about time constraints during a patient visit.[39]

There are situations that offer clinicians the opportunity to identify ACEs:

- A pediatrician can recognize when a child has been neglected or observed violence in the home;
- An emergency physician may treat an adolescent after a suicide attempt, assault, or drug overdose;
- An obstetrician may observe a sexually transmitted disease as an indication of sexual abuse;
- A family medicine provider can screen patients during a routine visit[40]; results are calculated quickly and the provider can discuss the outcomes immediately with the patient, if appropriate, with a minimal requirement of additional time.

SUMMARY

National initiatives are well-established that measure and guide prevention or mitigation of adversity in childhood. It is critical that the medical community makes it a priority to identify ACEs in children and adults. The clinician can and should offer treatment and/or social services that provide care or decrease the impact of ACEs for pediatric patients. Adults with a history of childhood trauma should receive care from mental health professionals.[41] Treatment may improve a clinician's ability to manage some of the serious sequalae that result from a history of childhood abuse. It is important for health care providers to link chronic disease or dangerous health behaviors in their adult patients to ACEs. An additional concern is that patients may not seek support services or may experience barriers to access support services.

Box 3 offers additional, subtopical references about ACEs.

Box 3	
Additional ACE publications by subtopic	
Childhood residential mobility and increased health risks	Dong et al,[42] 2005
Homelessness in childhood	Radcliff et al,[43] 2019
Intimate partner violence	Pro et al,[44] 20
Health care utilization	Koball et al,[45] 2019
	Grimes,[46] 2017
Increased risk of chronic diseases in adults who are deaf	Kushalnagar et al,[47] 2020
Suicidality in young people	Angelakis et al,[48] 2020
Suicidality in adults	Angelakis et al,[49] 2019
Sexual minorities	Andersen and Blosnich,[50] 2013
Decreased renal function	Ozieh et al,[51] 2020
Preventing ACEs	Centers for Disease Control and Prevention,[52] 2019

CLINICS CARE POINTS

- For many adults, ACEs are likely and are the result of adversity and trauma during childhood.

- Prevalence data for children and documented evidence of damage to biologic and behavioral systems point to the need to assess children for ACEs.

- ACEs can be present in children without evidence from a physical examination or other external signs of abuse and/or neglect.

- Children in low-income, rural homes are at higher risk for ACEs.

- ACEs can be intergenerational, and parents or guardians may abuse their children.

- Interview based screening tools are available to obtain a report about ACEs for a child from their parents or guardian.

- Public policy and national initiatives have prioritized ACEs as a public health problem and disseminate prevention strategies for implementation within clinical and community environments.

DISCLOSURE

The author has nothing to disclose.

REFERENCES

1. Bethell C, Newacheck P, Hawes E, et al. Adverse childhood experiences: addressing the impact on health and school engagement and the mitigating role of resilience. Health Aff 2014;33(12):2106–15.
2. Finkelhor D. Screening for adverse childhood experiences (ACES): cautions and suggestions. Child Abuse Negl 2018;85:175–9.
3. Felitti VJ, Anda R, Nordenberg D, et al. Relationship of childhood abuse and household dysfunction to many of the leading causes of death in adults: the adverse childhood experiences (ACE) Study. Am J Prev Med 1998;14(4):245–58.
4. Dube S. Twenty years and counting: the past, present, and future of ACEs research. In: Asmundson G, Afifi T, editors. Adverse childhood experiences: using evidence to advance research, Practice, policy, and prevention. Elsevier

Science & Technology; 2019. ProQuest Ebook Central, Available at: https://www.sciencedirect.com/science/article/pii/B978012816065700001X.

5. Bethell CD, Davis MB, Gombojav N, et al. Issue Brief: a national and across state profile on adverse childhood experiences among children and possibilities to heal and thrive. Baltimore: Johns Hopkins Bloomberg School of Public Health; 2017. Available at: http://www.cahmi.org/projects/adverse-childhood-experiences-aces/. Accessed November 16, 2020.

6. Kobita R, Tyrka A, Kelly M, et al. Interplay between childhood maltreatment, parental bonding, and gender effect: impact on quality of life. Child Abuse Negl 2008;32(1):19–34.

7. Felitti VJ. Childhood sexual abuse, depression, and family dysfunction in adult obese patients: a case control study. South Med J 1993;86(7):732–6.

8. Felitti VJ. Origins of the ACE Study. Am J Prev Med 2019;56(6):787–9.

9. Dong M, Anda R, Felitti V, et al. The interrelatedness of multiple forms of childhood abuse, neglect, and household dysfunction. Child Abuse Negl 2004; 28(7):771–84.

10. McGinnis JM, Foege WH. Actual causes of death in the United States. JAMA 1993;270:2207.

11. Hughes K, Bellis M, Hardcastle K, et al. The effect of multiple adverse childhood experiences on health: a systematic review and meta-analysis. Lancet Public Health 2017;2(8):e356–66.

12. Zarse E, Neff M, Yoder R, et al. The adverse childhood experiences questionnaire: two decades of research on childhood trauma as a primary cause of adult mental illness, addiction and medical diseases. Cogent Med 2019;6(1):2–24.

13. Lacey R, Minnis H. Practitioner review: twenty years of research with adverse childhood experience scores – Advantages, disadvantages and applications to practice. J Child Psychol Psychiatry 2020;61(2):116–30.

14. Kelly-Irving M, Delpierre C. A critique of the adverse childhood experiences framework in epidemiology and public health: uses and misuses. Soc Policy Soc. 2019;18(3):445–56.

15. Merrick MT, Ford DC, Ports KA, et al. Vital signs: estimated proportion of adult health problems attributable to adverse childhood experiences and implications for prevention — 25 States, 2015-2017. MMWR Morb Wkly Rep 2019;68(44): 999–1005.

16. Centers for Disease Control and Prevention. Behavioral Risk Factor Surveillance System survey ACE data, 2009-2018. Atlanta, GA: US Department of Health and Human Services Centers for Disease Control and Prevention; 2019.

17. Bethell C, Carle A, Hudziak J, et al. Methods to assess adverse childhood experiences of children and families: toward approaches to promote child well-being in policy and practice. Acad Pediatr 2017;17(7S):S51–69.

18. Crouch E, Probst J, Radcliff E, et al. Prevalence of adverse childhood experiences (ACEs) among US children. Child Abuse Negl 2019;92:209–18.

19. Merrick M, Ford D, Ports K, et al. Prevalence of adverse childhood experiences from the 2011-2014 Behavioral Risk Factor Surveillance System in 23 States. JAMA Pediatr 2018;172(11):1038–44.

20. LaBrenz C, Panisch L, Lawson J, et al. Adverse childhood experiences and outcomes among at-risk Spanish-speaking Latino families. J Child Fam Stud 2020; 29(5):1221–35.

21. Facts for features: Hispanic heritage month 2017. Census.gov. Available at: https://www.census.gov/content/dam/Census/newsroom/facts-for-features/2017/cb17-ff17.pdf. Accessed November 16, 2020.

22. Crouch E, Radcliff E, Probst J, et al. Rural-urban differences in adverse childhood experiences across a national sample of children. J Rural Health 2020;36(1): 55–64.
23. Kerker B, Zhang J, Nadeem E, et al. Adverse childhood experiences and mental health, chronic medical conditions and development in young children. Acad Pediatr 2015;15(5):510–7.
24. De Bellis M, Zisk A. The biological effects of childhood trauma. Child Adolesc Psychiatr Clin N Am 2014;23(2):185–222.
25. Ehlert U. Enduring psychobiological effects of childhood adversity. Psychoneruoendocrinology 2013;38(9):1850–7.
26. Jones D, Greenberg M, Crowley M. Early social-emotional functioning and public health: the relationship between kindergarten social competence and future wellness. Am J Public Health 2015;105(11):2283–90.
27. Szilagyi M, Halfon N. Pediatric adverse childhood experiences: Implications for life course health trajectories. Acad Pediatr 2015;15(5):467–8.
28. Shonkoff JP, Garner AS. Committee on Psychosocial Aspects of Child and Family Health; Committee on Early Childhood Adoption, and Dependent Care; Section on Developmental and Behavioral Pediatrics. The lifelong effects of early childhood adversity and toxic stress. Pediatrics 2012;129(1):e232–46.
29. McEwen BS. Stress, adaptation, and disease. Allostasis and allostatic load. Ann N Y Acad Sci 1998;840:33–44.
30. Campbell JA, Walker RJ, Egede LE. Associations between adverse childhood experiences, high-risk behaviors, and morbidity in adulthood. Am J Prev Med 2016; 50(3):344–52.
31. Edwards Anda R, Gu D, Dube S, et al. Adverse childhood experiences and smoking persistence in adults with smoking-related symptoms and illness. Perm J 2007;11(2):5–13.
32. Anda R, Croft J, Felitti V, et al. Adverse childhood experiences and smoking during adolescence and adulthood. JAMA 1999;282(17):1652–8.
33. Mersky JP, Topitzes J, Reynolds AJ. Impacts of adverse childhood experiences on health, mental health, and substance use in early adulthood: a cohort study of an urban, minority sample in the U.S. Child Abuse Negl 2013;37(11):917–25.
34. Fortson BL, Klevens J, Merrick MT, et al. Preventing child abuse and neglect: a technical package for policy, norm, and programmatic activities. Atlanta, GA: National Center for Injury Prevention and Control, Centers for Disease Control and Prevention; 2016. Available at: https://www.cdc.gov/violenceprevention/pdf/can-prevention-technical-package.pdf. Accessed November 16, 2020.
35. Centers for Disease Control and Prevention. Preventing adverse childhood experiences (ACES): leveraging the best available evidence. Atlanta, GA: National Center for Injury Prevention and Control, Centers for Disease Control and Prevention; 2019. Available at: https://www.cdc.gov/violenceprevention/pdf/preventingACES.pdf. Accessed November 16, 2020.
36. Marie-Mitchell A, Kostolansky R. A systematic review of trials to improve child outcomes associated with adverse childhood experiences. Am J Prev Med 2019; 56(5):756–64.
37. Jones C, Merrick M, Houry D. Identifying and preventing adverse childhood experiences: implications for clinical practice. JAMA 2020;323(1):25–6.
38. Flynn A, Fothergill K, Wilcox H, et al. Primary care interventions to prevent or treat traumatic stress in childhood: a systematic review. Acad Pediatr 2015;15(5): 480–92.

39. Esden JL. Adverse childhood experiences and implementing trauma-informed primary care. Nurse Pract 2018;43(12):10–21.

40. Glowa P, Olson A, Johnson D. Screening for adverse childhood experiences in a family medicine setting: a feasibility study. J Am Board Fam Med 2016;29(3): 303–7.

41. Korotana L, Dobson K, Pusch D, et al. A review of primary care interventions to improve health outcomes in adult survivors of adverse childhood experiences. Clin Psychol Rev 2016;46:59–90.

42. Dong M, Anda R, Felitti V, et al. Childhood residential mobility and multiple health risks during adolescence and adulthood. Arch Pediatr Adolesc Med 2005;159: 1104–10.

43. Radcliff E, Crouch E, Strompolis M, et al. Homelessness in childhood and adverse childhood experiences. Matern Child Health J 2019;23:811–20.

44. Pro G, Camplain R, de Heer B, et al. A national epidemiologic profile of physical intimate partner violence, adverse childhood experiences, and supportive childhood relationships: group differences in predicted trends and associations. J Racial Ethnic Health Disparities 2020;7:660–70.

45. Koball A, Rasmussen C, Olson-Dorff D, et al. The relationship between adverse childhood experiences, healthcare utilization, cost of care and medical comorbidities. Child Abuse Neglect 2019;90:120–6.

46. Grimes K. Lessons from ACEs: pay now or pay (more) later. Acad Pediatr 2017; 17:S18–9.

47. Kushalnaagar P, Ryan C, Paludneviciene R, et al. Adverse Childhood Communication Experiences Associated with An Increased Risk of Chronic Diseases in Adults who are Deaf. Am J Prev Med 2020;59:548–54.

48. Angelakis I, Austin J, Gooding P. Association of childhood maltreatment with suicide behaviors among young people: a systematic review and meta-analysis. JAMA Netw Open 2020;3:e2012563.

49. Angelakis I, Gillespie E, Panagioti M. Childhood maltreatment and adult suicidality: a comprehensive systematic review with meta-analysis. Psychol Med 2019; 49:1057–78.

50. Andersen J, Blosnich J. Disparities in adverse childhood experiences among sexual minority and heterosexual adults: results from a multi-state probability-based sample. PLoS One 2013;8(1):e54691.

51. Ozieh M, Garacci E, Campbell J, et al. Adverse childhood experiences and decreased renal function: impact on all-cause mortality in US Adults. Am J Prev Med 2020;59:e49–57.

52. Centers for Disease Control and Prevention. Preventing adverse childhood experiences: leveraging the best available evidence. Atlanta, GA: National Center for Injury Prevention and Control, Centers for Disease Control and Prevention; 2019.

Childhood Obesity

Neena Thomas-Eapen, MD

KEYWORDS

- Childhood obesity • Etiology • Complications • Healthy diet • Physical activity
- Pharmacotherapy • Bariatric surgery • Treatment

KEY POINTS

- Childhood obesity is a pathologic process with multifactorial causes: genetics, individual and family reasons, psycho socioeconomic reasons, organic pathology, and aftereffect of government policies.
- The list of complications of obesity in children is long and complicated: diabetes mellitus, hyperlipidemia, hypertension, and obstructive sleep apnea, to name a few.
- The management of obesity is multiprong, involving the patient, family, school, community, and even influencing policies.
- Lifestyle changes are the mainstay of treatment. Medications and bariatric surgery may have a role in certain severe cases.

INTRODUCTION

The World Health Organization defines overweight and obesity as abnormal or excessive fat accumulation that is risky to health. Obesity is one of the most severe public health problems of this century.[1]

Obesity in children has become a global epidemic and a serious public health challenge. It is a problem of the developed countries of the West as well as Asian and African countries. More than 41 million children younger than 5 years were overweight or obese globally, according to a 2016 study.[1] Children who are obese tend to remain obese through their childhood, putting them at risk for significant chronic diseases and complications.[1] Overweight and obesity are preventable causes that primary care physicians must identify and address.

In the United States, obesity in children and adolescents is a major medical issue that puts them at high mortality and morbidity in their adult lives. Among the pediatric population of 2 to 19 years, 18.5% is the prevalence of obesity, which means that approximately 13.7 million children and adolescents are affected by obesity. Hispanic individuals have the highest prevalence of 25.8%, followed by non-Hispanic black individuals with 22%. Non-Hispanic white individuals have a lower prevalence of 14.1%. Non-Hispanic Asian individuals have the lowest prevalence of 11%. As the education

College of Medicine, University of Kentucky, 2195 Harrodsburg Road, Suite 125, Lexington, KY 4005-3504, USA
E-mail address: neena.thomas@uky.edu

Prim Care Clin Office Pract 48 (2021) 505–515
https://doi.org/10.1016/j.pop.2021.04.002
0095-4543/21/© 2021 Elsevier Inc. All rights reserved.

level of the household increased, the obesity prevalence decreased. Obesity was highest among middle-income children (19.9%) and lowest among the highest-income groups (10.9%). The lowest income group also has a significant prevalence of 18.9%.[2]

DEFINITION

Body mass index (BMI) is a person's weight in kilograms divided by the square of height in meters. BMI can be correlated with other direct body measures, even though it does not measure body fat.[2]

BMI is easily calculated from the Centers for Disease Control and Prevention (CDC) Web site link: https://www.cdc.gov/healthyweight/bmi/calculator.html.[2]

Compared with children and teens of the same age and sex, overweight is at or above the 85th percentile. Obesity is at or above the 95th percentile. Underweight is less than the fifth percentile. Normal weight is from 5th to 85th percentile.[2–5]

RELEVANCE

Childhood obesity predicts adult obesity. Fifty percent of the girls and 30% of boys who are obese between age 6 years and 11 years will be obese adults, predisposing themselves to chronic medical issues over the years. Sixty percent of obese adolescents remain obese as adults. Children with obesity tend to have morbid obesity in adulthood more than those who become obese as adults.[6]

PREDICTORS AND ETIOLOGY

The best predictor for childhood obesity is parental obesity. If children have one obese parent, the children tend to have adult obesity. Parental obesity predicts future obesity in a child younger than 3 years, more than the child's weight.[6]

The obesity epidemic has multifactorial causes, including biological, psychological, environmental, and societal factors. The human body stores energy in adipose tissue as a reserve for survival in case of famine. Even small sustained incremental excess calories add on to fat tissue.[7] At the basic level, obesity is an imbalance of intake of calories and expenditure of energy. Less energy use by physical activities and excess calorie intake from food and drinks by quantity or frequency leads to obesity.[7]

The time from conception to 2 years of age for the child can be modified to influence childhood obesity. Breastfeeding gives moderate protection to prevent obesity depending on the frequency and duration.[7] Maternal factors predisposing to pediatric obesity are maternal diabetes, maternal smoking, and gestational weight gain.[8] Rapid infant growth also is a risk for future obesity.

Lifestyle and societal changes are the main reasons for the rise in obesity in the past 20 years. Genetic factors only play a small role in obesity.[6]

The lifestyle changes that led to the obesity epidemic are as follows[7]:

Lack of home-cooked whole food meals.

Use of industrially prepared high-calorie processed foods.

Use of foods that are high on simple, refined carbohydrates and added sugar.

Regular use of high-carbohydrate beverages with empty calories like sodas, sports drinks, punches, and juices.

Use of high-fructose corn syrup to mass-produce inexpensive sweetened beverages and foods that are readily available.

Regular consumption of fast foods that are cheap but packed with high calories and unhealthy fats.

Table 1 Endocrine causes of pediatric obesity	
Cushing syndrome	Growth hormone deficiency
Hyperinsulinism	Hypothyroidism
Pseudohypoparathyroidism	

Increased snacking between meals, mainly processed snacks.

Larger portion sizes.

Marketing pressure and advertisements.

Decreased physical activity and sedentary life.

Increased screen time.

Unsafe neighborhoods to go out and safely play.

Budget constraints of the family.

The fast pace of life preventing from cooking at home and eating together at the dining table.

Decreased sleeping time, causing sleep debt.

In a small number of cases, a hormonal imbalance may be the etiology of obesity. Endocrine causes include the following:

Table 1 gives a list of endocrine pathologies that need to be considered in the clinical examination and workup of obesity.[7]

Genetics

Mutations and abnormalities of genes can lead to obesity. **Table 2** gives the list of the syndromes that can be associated with obesity.[7]

Gut Microbiome

There is mounting evidence that the gut microbiome plays a significant role in regulating metabolism and disruption, causing obesity.[9] Frequent use of unnecessary

Table 2 Genetic causes of pediatric obesity	
Albright hereditary osteodystrophy	Alstrom syndrome
Bardet- Biedl syndrome	BDNF/TrkB deficiency
Biemond syndrome	Carpenter syndrome
Cohen syndrome	Deletion 9q34
Down Syndrome	ENPP1 gene mutations
Frohlich syndrome	FTO gene polymorphism
KSR2 deficiency	Leptin or leptin receptor gene deficiency
Melanocortin 4 receptor gene mutation	PCSK1 deficiency
Prader-Willi syndrome	Proopiomelanocortin (POMC) deficiency
Rapid-onset obesity with hypothalamic dysfunction, hypoventilation, and autonomic dysregulation (ROHHAD)	SH2B1 deficiency
SIM1 deficiency	TUB deficiency
Turner syndrome	

antibiotics may cause a shift in intestinal bacterial flora. Hence, it is essential to avoid prescribing antibiotics when not indicated, such as in viral infections. It is also important to consistently include fiber-rich, nutrient-dense foods, including prebiotics and fermented foods containing probiotics, to keep a healthy gut microbiome.

Neuroendocrine Physiology

Short-term control of satiety and appetite happens through complex neuroendocrine feedback loops through adipose tissue, gastrointestinal system, and central nervous system. Many hormones are involved in this complex cycle, like cholecystokinin, glucagonlike peptide-1, peptide YY, and vagal neuronal peptide, promoting satiety. Ghrelin stimulates appetite. Leptin is another crucial hormone. Low levels of leptin increase food intake.[7]

Medications Associated with Obesity

Children and adolescents may be on prescription medications for various physical or mental illnesses. If there is rapid weight gain in a short period, these medications need to be discontinued or adjusted. The common pharmaceuticals associated with weight gain and obesity are prednisone and other glucocorticoids, thioridazine, olanzapine, clozapine, quetiapine, risperidone, lithium, amitriptyline, and other tricyclic antidepressants, paroxetine, valproate, carbamazepine, gabapentin, cyproheptadine, propranolol, and other β-blockers.[7]

COMORBIDITIES AND COMPLICATIONS

Obesity is a major medical issue due to its adverse effects or comorbidities. Many of these complications are not part of a normal childhood in children and adolescents without a genetic cause or endocrine cause. However, the obesity epidemic has put many pediatric populations at risk for these chronic diseases of lifestyle with long-term complications. The list in **Table 3** gives the possible common complications of obesity under different systems.[7]

Table 3	
Adverse effects and complications of pediatric obesity	
Cardiovascular	Dyslipidemia, hypertension
Endocrine	Diabetes mellitus type 2, metabolic syndrome, polycystic ovarian syndrome
Gastrointestinal	Gallbladder disease, nonalcoholic fatty liver disease
Neurologic	Pseudotumor cerebri, migraine
Mental health	Anxiety, depression, low self-esteem, worsening school performance, social isolation, problems of bullying
Orthopedic	Tibia vara, back pain, joint pain, strains, and sprains, slipped capital femoral epiphysis
Pulmonary	Obstructive sleep apnea, asthma
Oncology	Breast, colon, and endometrial cancer; there is an increased risk of these malignancies as obesity continues to adulthood
Chronic inflammation	The adipose tissue releases peptides and cytokines into the circulation, acting as a secretory organ causing low-grade chronic inflammation in the body[6]

SCREENING

The US Preventive Services Task Force (USPSTF) recommends (Level B) BMI as the measure of obesity.[8] This is plotted during routine child and adolescent wellness examinations. Obesity is diagnosed based on the CDC-recommended BMI graphs. Age-specific and sex-specific BMI in the 95th percentile or greater is obesity.[8,10]

The USPSTF found no evidence regarding appropriate screening intervals for obesity in children and adolescents, but it is expected that the BMI is calculated at regular visits and addressed if needed by pediatric experts. The USPSTF did not find sufficient evidence on screening in children younger than 6 years. Evidence of effective interventions in children younger than 6 years is limited.[8] Effective behavioral interventions were targeted at children 6 years and older.[10,11] Pediatric experts believe that early recognition and early intervention are the keys to curbing the condition's progress and its morbidity successfully.[7]

EVALUATION

During routine visits for health maintenance or wellness examinations, assess the BMI. According to the CDC criteria for age and gender, If the BMI Is high, assess further.[7]

1. Anthropometric data: measure the height and weight and calculate BMI. Determine the percentage according to CDC graphs matching for age and gender to see whether it is in a range of overweight or obesity.
2. Once obesity is determined, take a diet history and family history to understand the patient's behavioral habits, family dynamics, routines, and customs.
3. Explore the details about physical activity and screen time.
4. A thorough physical examination will help to point toward endocrine or genetic epidemiology, which may need further workup.
5. Look for complications due to obesity and comorbidities.
6. Do necessary workup and investigations to diagnose or screen common adverse effects of obesity as appropriately directed by history and physical for hyperlipidemia, diabetes, obstructive sleep apnea, or other problems as given in the previous list. Nine-year-olds to 11-year-olds need a lipid screen. Other laboratory tests may include blood glucose, glycosylated hemoglobin, and liver function tests. If indicated, order a home sleep study or overnight oxygen monitoring to evaluate obstructive sleep apnea.
7. Ask the patient and family whether they are willing to discuss the obesity and weight problem and whether they are ready to make changes.
8. Motivational interviewing with reflective listening and open-ended questions may help determine the reasons, barriers to change, and motivate patients and families to make the positive changes.[12]

INTERVENTIONS, GOALS, AND TREATMENT

According to USPSTF, 26 hours of comprehensive, intense behavioral interventions over 2 to 12 months resulted in weight loss.[8,11,13] More than 52 contact hours resulted in more weight loss.

Successful interventions include the following: information about healthy foods and eating habits, stimulus control, food label reading, not having tempting foods, goal setting, self-monitoring, contingent rewards, limiting screen time, problem-solving, and supervised physical activity sessions. Fifty-two-hour sessions were done by multidisciplinary teams, including pediatricians, exercise physiologists or physical therapists, dieticians or diet assistants, psychologists or social workers, or other behavioral specialists.[8,9,11]

Whatever changes are made in diet, physical activity, and behavior must be long-term, as obesity is a lifelong chronic medical issue. The interventions and treatments need to continue lifelong as in any other chronic disease state like hypertension and diabetes. Patients and families need to understand it.

In growing young individuals, the goal is to make adequate diet and physical activity changes with the family's help to maintain the weight to grow closer to a weight normal for their height.[11]

There are 2 approaches to diet prescription. One approach is to prescribe a 1300-calorie to 1500-calorie diet to girls and a 1500-calorie to 1800-calorie diet to boys. The alternate approach is to prescribe a diet with a calorie deficit of 500 to 750 calories per day calculated for the beginning weight and recalculate the permitted calories based on the new weight as obesity improves. Commercial weight loss programs are challenging to sustain. Very low-calorie diets are also difficult to follow.[11]

Increased physical activity through activities of daily living or structured programs is essential. To achieve it, children and adolescents need to cut down screen time. The new digital technology and devices may help count the steps, energy spending, counting calories, and monitoring goal achievement.

Those who cannot achieve significant weight loss by these measures need to be referred for intense behavioral counseling with a trained therapist.[7] The patients need to be trained to do small, incremental, and consistent positive changes. In-person, high-intensity, comprehensive behavioral counseling results in more successful weight loss.[7]

PHARMACOTHERAPY

Certain selected patients with severe obesity or lower obesity with multiple comorbidities may be candidates for pharmacotherapy.[7,8] Two main medications are used for pediatric obesity.[7,11] Other medicines have been studied in small studies. Medications are reserved for patients with comorbidities or for those who are not successful with diet and behavioral interventions.

1. Orlistat is approved to be used in children older than 12 years. It has only a small effect on weight loss.[14] It is the only medication approved by the Food and Drug Administration (FDA) to treat pediatric obesity. It is an inhibitor of pancreatic lipase and lipase that limits the absorption of dietary fat.[15] The dose is 120 mg up to 3 times a day with meals containing fat, or less than 1 hour after meals. *Average weight loss with the medicine for a 100-kg patient was −6.1%.*[7] If the meal is skipped or does not have fat, the dose can be missed. There was a modest improvement in weight with orlistat when combined with lifestyle therapy.[16] Gastrointestinal side effects are the main adverse effects.[14] These include flatulence, oily stools, and spotting. However, if strict instructions about reduced fat intake and a healthy diet are followed, the side effects will be less. It can cause decreased absorption of fat-soluble vitamins like A, D, E, and K. Hence, prescribe multivitamins daily. It should be taken 2 hours before or after the orlistat.
2. Metformin is used in children in some studies. It has a small effect on weight loss. It is not approved for use by the FDA for the treatment of childhood obesity. However, doctors have a lot of experience with metformin in young adults to treat diabetes mellitus and polycystic ovary syndrome. It is a relatively safe drug. The dose is 500 mg to 1000 mg up to twice a day in children older than 10 years.[17] It is an anti-hyperglycemic agent that is indicated for the treatment of type 2 diabetes mellitus.

It decreases hepatic glucose production, reduces intestinal absorption of glucose, and improves insulin sensitivity by increasing peripheral glucose uptake and utilization. It does not cause hypoglycemia.[7]

3. Other pharmacologic agents studied include exenatide and topiramate.[15] The FDA approves none for use in weight loss in children and adolescents.

4. Liraglutide is a glucagonlike peptide 1 analog. It was used in a trial for weight loss and had a more significant BMI reduction (−4.64% change in BMI in Liraglutide group) than placebo with lifestyle therapy. However, this is not FDA approved for this indication in the pediatric age group.[18]

5. Hormone replacement therapy is an emerging pharmacotherapy for specific cases with leptin receptor deficiency. Setmelanotide activates MC_4R (melanocortin 4 receptor) and binds to it. This is a useful emerging therapy for obese patients with proopiomelanocortin deficiency.[19]

BARIATRIC SURGERY AND ENDOSCOPIC PROCEDURES

Invasive surgeries and procedures may be a last resort reserved for adolescents. Roux-en-Y gastric bypass surgery is the most common one performed. Other surgeries in the pipeline include vertical sleeve gastrectomy and adjustable gastric band procedure.[20]

The criteria for candidate selection for bariatric surgery are as follows:

1. Adolescents with a BMI of 35 kg/m^2 or higher with significant comorbidities like diabetes mellitus type 2, moderate to severe sleep apnea, and severe nonalcoholic fatty liver disease.

2. Adolescents with a BMI of 40 kg/m^2 or higher with significant comorbidities like hypertension, dyslipidemia, impaired quality of life, or sleep apnea.

3. Others recommend stricter criteria of BMI of 40 to 50 kg/m^2 or higher in the presence of comorbidities.

The patients must meet additional criteria of final or near-final attainment of adult height determined by pubertal development or bone age, failure of organized weight loss attempt for 12 months, supportive family environment, and emotional and cognitive maturity.

Surgery must be performed at a bariatric center of excellence with special expertise in adolescent patients. Outcomes in adolescents are comparable to adults and sometimes even better.[20]

Contraindications for surgical procedures include preadolescent child, unresolved eating disorders, Prader-Willi syndrome, pregnancy, breastfeeding, plan to become pregnant within 2 years, and untreated psychiatric disorder.[21]

Bariatric surgery complications can include anastomotic stricture, gastrointestinal leak, small bowel obstruction, dumping syndrome, and nutritional deficiencies due to malabsorption.

PREVENTION

There are 3 levels of prevention.[7]

Primordial prevention is keeping normal weight for height throughout childhood and adolescence.

Primary prevention is taking measures to prevent overweight children from becoming obese.

Secondary prevention is taking measures to prevent comorbidities in obese children and adolescents and reverse obesity and overweight if possible.

Multiple interventions in the long term are the only solution for reducing the obesity epidemic. Multiple strategies can be done on a personal, family, health care system, community, and government level to reduce obesity in the population.[7]

Exclusive breastfeeding for the first 6 months of life has a protective effect on the prevention of obesity later in life.[7]

During pregnancy, the following strategies can help:

- Normalize BMI before pregnancy.
- Do not smoke.
- Maintain moderate exercise as tolerated.
- In women with gestational diabetes, provide meticulous glucose control.
- Keep gestational weight gain within recommendations.

Strategies that help during the first year of life:

- Breastfeeding exclusively for 4 to 6 months; continue breastfeeding with other foods for 12 months.
- Postpone introduction of baby foods to 4 to 6 months and juices to 12 months.

On an individual level during the latter years, these are the strategies that can help:

Physical activity more than an hour a day from activities of daily living or designated exercise time.

Limited screen time less than 1 to 2 hours per day. No screen time for those younger than 2 years. This includes television, computer games, video games, smartphone.

Consume at least 5, if possible, 8 servings of vegetables and fruits per day.

Include prebiotic foods such as apples, leeks, onions, bananas, garlic, asparagus, artichokes, barley, oats, wheat bran, and sea algae.

Include fermented foods for probiotics, such as plain yogurt, kefir, sauerkraut, miso, pickles, traditional buttermilk from yogurt, and small amounts of cheeses like cheddar, mozzarella, gouda (not more than the size of a domino per day).

No added sugar-sweetened beverages or juices.

Healthy whole food for breakfast daily.

Never eat from a bag.

Use smaller bowls and plates.

Learn about satiety cues.

The strategies a family can implement include the following:

Have meals at a table as a family at least 5 to 6 times per week.

Prepare whole food meals at home.

Freeze extra home-cooked meals so that healthy meals are available when needed.

Make eating out and purchasing from a restaurant very occasional, less than once a week.

Allow the child to self-regulate his or her meals.

Do not insist on finishing all the food on the plate.

Do not give food and drinks as incentives.

Provide healthy snacks like fruits, nuts, seeds, vegetables.

Avoid serving sweets and desserts regularly.

Allow occasional treats in smaller portion sizes.

Keep children involved in shopping for healthy ingredients, cooking, storing, and cleaning in the kitchen.

Always encourage outdoor activities.

Keep children busy with healthy activities.

Do outside physical activities together as a family like hiking, riding bikes, dancing, and visiting a zoo.

Encourage walking with a friend and talking rather than talking over the phone.

Buy active toys more than video games and videos.

Enroll children in swimming, martial arts, and sports.

These are measures health care workers and clinicians can provide:

Take a few minutes to take a nutrition history, which may reveal high-risk areas.

Speak to patients and families about home-cooked whole food meals and physical activity.

Make appropriate referrals and point toward the right resources.

Work with community centers like extension centers and schools to educate on a healthy diet and physical activity.

Measures schools can take include the following:

Serve healthy whole foods.

Serve a whole food high-protein breakfast.

Do not stock sodas, juices, juice beverages, processed high fat, refined starchy food in vending machines. Stock water, flavored water, sparkling water, fruits, nuts and seeds, vegetables, and whole-grain high-protein snacks.

Have an outdoor recess.

Have a home economics class to teach children about healthy choices, healthy grocery shopping, cooking, and food storage.

Provide education classes for parents and children together.

Avoid candy, cookies, processed food, and beverage sales as fundraisers.

Avoid candy and processed starchy goods as a reward by teachers in the classrooms.

Avoid fund support for sports teams from food and beverage companies.

Mandate 60 minutes of physical education class 5 days a week.

Provide education on a healthy diet, physical activity, and healthy lifestyle from kindergarten to high school for all children.

Government/Policy Can Make Long-Term Positive Effects on Obesity Prevention

Increase access to healthy whole foods.

Regulate food for healthy nutrition and smaller serving sizes.

Make regulations about nutrition labels so that people can understand it easily.

Regulate food advertisements.

Work on subsidies given for cash crops to nutrition-dense vegetables, fruits, nuts, seeds, beans, lentils, and healthy proteins.

Plan more sidewalks and parks to encourage walking and biking.

Have more facilities for public transport.

Make facilities for free or subsidized physical activities.

Ban toys with fast food.

Incentivize to make communities with residential and business complexes so that people can walk around to get things done.

FINAL THOUGHTS

Many present-generation young children and adolescents may not outlive their parents or grandparents due to obesity-related chronic medical problems and their complications. Unless we work together as a team from the government to the individual level involving all people, we will not reduce the obesity epidemic and reduce complications. The obesity epidemic will drive health care costs up. Filling society with unhealthy members adds burden at multiple levels, and affects the nation's and world's health. Hence, this health crisis needs immediate attention to reduce the prevalence, incidence, morbidity, and mortality.

CLINICS CARE POINTS

- The USPSTF recommends screening for obesity in children 6 years and older and offer or refer them to comprehensive, intensive behavioral interventions to improve weight. Grade B recommendation.
- Pediatric specialists recommend checking BMI during routine visits to identify overweight and obesity based on the CDC graphs.
- BMI more than 85% is overweight, and more than 95% is obesity in children and adolescents for age-matched and sex-matched data compared with the CDC weight and height graphs.
- Endocrine causes are infrequent in the etiology of childhood obesity.
- Environmental factors interact with genetic factors to cause obesity.
- A combination of healthy diet interventions for height, daily regular physical activity, and behavior change makes the weight close to normal.
- Pharmacotherapy and bariatric surgery are useful in severely obese adolescents.
- Orlistat is the only FDA-approved medical therapy for the pediatric population older than 12 years.
- Bariatric surgery is reserved for very severe obesity or moderate obesity with complications.
- Breastfeeding for the first 6 months of life significantly reduces obesity in the future.
- Family support is essential in the treatment.
- Schools, community resources, and town planning to incorporate physical activity into daily life and government policies make long-term improvements in the obesity epidemic.

DISCLOSURE

Nothing to disclose.

REFERENCES

1. Available at: https://www.who.int/news-room/q-a-detail/noncommunicable-diseases-childhood-overweight-and-obesity. Accessed December 21, 2020.
2. Available at: https://www.cdc.gov/obesity/data/childhood.html. Accessed December 21, 2020.
3. Barlow SE, the Expert Committee. Expert committee recommendations regarding the prevention, assessment, and treatment of child and adolescent overweight and obesity: summary report. Pediatrics 2007;120(Suppl 4):S164–92.
4. Cote AT, Harris KC, Panagiotopoulos C, et al. Childhood obesity and cardiovascular dysfunction. J Am Coll Cardiol 2013;62(15):1309–19.
5. Whitlock EP, Williams SB, Gold R, et al. Screening and interventions for childhood overweight: a summary of evidence for the US Preventive Services Task Force. Pediatrics 2005;116(1):e125–44.
6. McInerny TK, Adam HM, Campbell DE, et al. American Academy of Pediatrics textbook of pediatric care. Elk Grove Village (IL): American Academy of Pediatrics; 2016. p. 2396–406. Chapter 298.
7. Kliegman RM, Geme JSt. Nelson textbook of pediatrics. Elsevier; 2019. p. 345–60. Chapter 60.
8. Available at: https://www.uspreventiveservicestaskforce.org/uspstf/document/RecommendationStatementFinal/obesity-in-children-and-adolescents-screening. Accessed December 21, 2020.

9. Riva A, Borgo F, Lassandro C, et al. Pediatric obesity is associated with an altered gut microbiota and discordant shifts in Firmicutes populations. Environ Microbiol 2017;19(1):95–105.

10. Eder M, Lozano P. Screening for obesity and intervention for weight management in children and adolescents: evidence report and systematic review for the US Preventive Services Task Force. JAMA 2017;317(23):2427–44.

11. O'Connor EA, Evans CV, Burda BU, et al. Screening for obesity and intervention for weight management in children and adolescents: a systematic evidence review for the U.S. Preventive Services Task Force. Evidence synthesis No. 150. AHRQ Publication No. 15-05219-EF-1. Rockville (MD): Agency for Healthcare Research and Quality; 2017.

12. Huang JS, Barlow SE, Quiros-Tejeira RE, et al. Childhood obesity for pediatric gastroenterologists. J Pediatr Gastroenterol Nutr 2013;56(1):99–109.

13. O'Connor EA, Evans CV, Burda BU, et al. Screening and treatment for obesity in children and adolescents: systematic evidence review and evidence report for the U.S. Preventive Services Task Force recommendation statement. JAMA 2017;317(23):2427–44.

14. Available at: https://www.accessdata.fda.gov/drugsatfda_docs/label/2009/020766s026lbl.pdf. Accessed November 10, 2020.

15. Boland CL, Harris JB, Harris KB. Pharmacological management of obesity in pediatric patients. Ann Pharmacother 2015;49(2):220–32.

16. Matson KL, Fallon RM. Treatment of obesity in children and adolescents. J Pediatr Pharmacol Ther 2012;17(1):45–57.

17. Available at: https://www.accessdata.fda.gov/drugsatfda_docs/label/2017/020357s037s039,021202s021s023lbl.pdf. Accessed November 10, 2020.

18. Kelly AS, Auerbach P, Barrientos-Perez M, et al. A randomized, controlled trial of liraglutide for adolescents with obesity. N Engl J Med 2020;382(22):2117–28.

19. Clément K, Biebermann H, Farooqi IS, et al. MC4R agonism promotes durable weight loss in patients with leptin receptor deficiency. Nat Med 2018;24(5):551–5.

20. Michalsky M, Reichard K, Inge T, et al, American Society for Metabolic and Bariatric Surgery. ASMBS pediatric committee best practice guidelines. Surg Obes Relat Dis 2012;8(1):1–7.

21. Styne DM, Arslanian SA, Connor EL, et al. Pediatric obesity-assessment, treatment, and prevention: an endocrine society clinical practice guideline. J Clin Endocrinol Metab 2017;102(3):709–57.

Pediatric Allergy
An Overview

Check for updates

Arezoo Rajaee, MD, Meghane E. Masquelin, DO,
Katherine M. Pohlgeers, MD*

KEYWORDS

- Allergic rhinitis • Anaphylaxis • Atopic dermatitis • Chronic cough
- Contact dermatitis • Food allergy • Pediatric allergy • Urticaria

KEY POINTS

- Cow's milk, egg, wheat, and peanut are the most common pediatric allergens among which only peanut allergy is the most likely not to be outgrown.
- Food allergy is an adverse reproducible multisystem immune response, on exposure to a food. Food intolerance is a nonimmunologic metabolic response due to enzyme deficiencies.
- Allergic rhinitis makes up around 50% of all cases of rhinitis in the pediatric population.
- Environmental allergens induce allergen-specific immunoglobulin E (IgE), which is often transient and resolves spontaneously. Persistence and consolidation of such reactions leads to the development of allergies.
- Anaphylaxis is caused by degranulation of mast cells and systemic release of IgE complexes in response to an allergen, including food, drugs, and insect bites.

INTRODUCTION

The term "allergy" refers to an abnormal immunologic reaction on exposure to an allergen. Immunoglobulin E (IgE) antibodies produced against specific protein "allergens" activate mast cells and basophils. Other cellular processes involving eosinophils or T cells will also mediate allergic reactions.[1] Allergic disorders are driven by a complex interplay of a large number of leukocytes (especially mast cells, eosinophils, neutrophils, lymphocytes, basophils, dendritic cells [DC], innate lymphocytes, and lymphoid cells) and structural tissue cells (such as epithelial cells and fibroblasts).[2] Strictly regulated immune system of the mucosal surface prevents inappropriate immune reactions to food antigens or the commensal flora and is responsible for guarding a vast surface area against pathogenic entry.[3] This system activates a tolerance response when a pathogen gains access to the system, mediated by regulatory

Department of Family Medicine and Geriatrics, University of Louisville, 201 Abraham Flexner Way, Suite 690, Louisville, KY 40202, USA
* Corresponding author.
E-mail address: katherine.pohlgeers@louisville.edu

Prim Care Clin Office Pract 48 (2021) 517–530
https://doi.org/10.1016/j.pop.2021.04.006
0095-4543/21/© 2021 Elsevier Inc. All rights reserved.

T cells and induced by gastrointestinal DCs and macrophages. Consistently, the 2 critical factors in the maintenance of gastrointestinal immune homeostasis are microbiota and diet.[4]

Allergic reactions are unique in that one allergic condition is often a risk factor for other similar diseases. They show higher prevalence in cities compared with suburbs and rural areas across the planet. The exception is the US inner cities where the prevalence of allergic diseases is particularly high.[5] Epidemiologists attribute this finding to the interaction of several environmental and genetic factors with no conclusive explanation for the rising trends. Geneticists have recently isolated several loci that seem to alter the susceptibility of an individual to allergic disease. Their studies have significantly contributed to our current understanding of these conditions. Exploring the complex epigenetic influences on allergic disease development and pathogenesis is likely the future orientation of allergy research. Consistently, children with underlying deficiency of host defense need to be identified by an allergist and be screened for such disorders.[6] On the other hand, environmental risk factors, such as exposure to daycare or cigarette smoke, are present in most of the children with recurrent respiratory tract infections associated with atopy.[7]

Allergy is a broad topic encompassing common clinical allergic diseases, asthma, and complex immunodeficiencies. Because of the breadth of the 2 latter topics, the authors have decided to discuss asthmatic diseases and immunodeficiencies in separate chapters. In this article they discuss the most common allergic diseases and anaphylaxis.

TYPES OF ALLERGENS
Outdoor Allergens

Airborne allergens originate from numerous sources with significant variation in size, ranging from bacteria, protozoa, and dust mites to mushrooms, cats, and dogs. They shed allergen deposits on conjunctival, nasal, pharyngeal, or pulmonary epithelial surfaces. This does not necessarily cause an allergic reaction or an infection.[8] An important factor in pathogenesis of airborne allergens is the volume and concentration of inoculation. Temperature and precipitation have the greatest impact on timing and intensity of airborne pollen concentration. Allergenic plants and pollen production increase with temperature and carbon dioxide concentration. Plants are the frequent source of outdoor allergens, whereas animal allergens are the origin of indoor ones; fungal spores are a source for both indoor and outdoor allergens.[9]

Indoor Allergens

Early life environmental exposure to a specific indoor allergen influences its sensitization and clinical atopic presentation. High humidity promotes house dust mite growth, which in turn may cause asthma.[10] More than 80% of school age children with asthma in inner cities and suburban locations are sensitized to at least one indoor allergen. For instance, several studies have demonstrated a relationship between cockroach exposure and higher asthma morbidity in children in urban settings. Because of lack of scientific evidence, current guidelines do not recommend hypoallergenic cats and dogs for those sensitized.[11]

MOST COMMON ALLERGIC DISEASE
Food Allergy

A food allergy is an adverse reproducible immune response involving skin, respiratory, gastrointestinal, or cardiovascular system, on exposure to a food protein.[12] Food intolerance, on the other hand, is a nonimmunologic response mostly of metabolic nature such as digestive enzyme deficiencies. Food allergies are either IgE mediated occurring within a few minutes of exposure in the skin, gastrointestinal tract, and lungs or are non–IgE mediated involving delayed reactions typically isolated to gastrointestinal tracts.[13]

Food allergies mostly claim themselves during infancy and early childhood causing a range of feeding disorders. In young children, food allergies commonly exacerbate atopic dermatitis and eczema symptoms. This age range may also present with feeding disorders due to eosinophilic esophagitis. Older patients on the other hand present with dysphagia, abdominal pain, frequent nausea and vomiting, diarrhea, and malabsorption.[14] Among the most common ones, cow milk allergies, for instance, often involve 2 or more organ systems.[15]

Dietary proteins may cause proctocolitis, enterocolitis, and enteropathy (including celiac disease). These allergic enteropathics represent cell-mediated hypersensitivity disorders, the symptoms of which generally present in infancy.[13] The immunologic mechanism of allergic enteropathies is not completely clear. The management is, however, simplified in either reintroduction of the food for tolerance assessment or prolonged elimination of the allergen from diet. Recently, the eosinophilic gastrointestinal disorders are becoming increasingly recognized.[16] Although gastric involvement is rare and difficult to diagnose, the pharyngeal and esophageal variants are much more common and easily diagnosed by endoscopic biopsy. It is not clear if the eosinophil dysregulation is caused by an immunologic defect or an allergy. Close collaboration of gastroenterologists, allergists, and dietitians is likely to shed more light on the pathogenesis and management of these enteropathies. Families may find it difficult to adopt restricted diets, which highlights the importance of establishing a system of support for this patient population.[17]

Oral allergy syndrome (OAS), also known as pollen food allergy syndrome, is an IgE-mediated food allergy resulting from cross-reactivities between plant pollens and homologous plant proteins. This syndrome is mostly mild and limited to the oropharynx, but systemic reactions have been reported.[18] OAS prevalence significantly varies across the globe, and it is generally managed by allergen abstinence. It is mostly associated with ingesting fresh fruits and vegetables. The heated food forms of the allergens are often well tolerated, which suggests the triggering proteins are heat-labile proteins.[19]

Once more, a thorough and detailed history is the most important part of the diagnosis. Skin tests and IgE levels confirm sensitization but are not enough evidence to establish diagnosis of clinical allergy, and the gold standard for diagnosing food allergy remains to be an oral food challenge. Controlled elimination/challenge tests are only able to confirm diagnosis in about one-third of the cases. Clinicians should always rule out normal food reactions before undertaking comprehensive diagnostic procedures.[20]

Allergic Rhinitis

Allergic rhinitis presents with nasal symptoms including sneezing, runny nose, nasal obstruction, and postnasal drainage, whereas the patient does not have a cold or flu and itching of the eyes, nose, and palate. Systemic symptoms including fatigue, irritability, decreased function affecting school and work, and depression can be found in some patients with more severe symptoms.[21] Allergic rhinitis prevalence is 10% to 30% in children and adults in the United States. Its prevalence is increasing in developed countries, affecting mostly the urban areas. Allergic rhinitis makes up around 50% of all cases of rhinitis in the pediatric population. Yet this disease is often overlooked in clinical settings.[22] Allergic rhinitis is classified as seasonal, perennial, or mixed based on timing and duration of allergen exposure. As the allergic rhinitis diagnosis is clinical, clinicians should be familiar with the signs and symptoms of the disease in children, especially of its main comorbidities, such as asthma, sinusitis, and otitis media, for a successful diagnosis and treatment plan and be familiar with differential diagnosis of allergic rhinitis (including acute and chronic rhinosinusitis [CRS], atrophic rhinitis, chronic nonallergic rhinitis, rhinitis medicamentosa, and rhinitis due to systemic medications) in order to make timely referral for specific testing.[23] If indicated, the diagnosis may be confirmed by presence of allergen-specific IgE, and exposure to the specific allergen should reproduce the symptoms. Apart from avoiding the allergen, treatment includes nonsedating antihistamines, nasal steroids, and immunotherapy.[24]

Otitis Media

Otitis media (OM) may be acute, chronic, or recurrent mainly caused by infections and Eustachian tube obstruction. OM with effusion (OME) is the most prevalent pediatric ear disease and the most common reason of acquired hearing impairment in children.[25] Allergic rhinitis plays a crucial role in the pathogenesis and the clinical picture, especially in more severe chronic or recurrent OM. OME and acute otitis media (AOM) are the 2 main subtypes of OM. Although OME is the middle ear effusion without infection, acute bacterial infection of the middle ear in AOM involves 70% of the cases. Given the high prevalence of these conditions, clinicians should become competent in differentiating AOM from OME.[26] Management of such patients will include consulting allergist-immunologists, otolaryngologists, and audiologists when indicated. Treatment should include a careful risk benefit consideration. It is of paramount importance to address the associated comorbidities and to identify children at risk for language delays. Because OM often presents with rhinitis, in chronic cases, it is important to determine whether this rhinitis is of infectious or allergic cause.[27] An allergic process presents as prolonged, perennial, or recurrent seasonal rhinitis where sneezing, pruritus, and conjunctivitis are seen. Presence of a family or personal history of allergy, atopy, asthma, and food allergies further substantiate an allergic cause. Pediatric patients with persistent OME should be screened for allergies and referred to an allergist for further diagnostic studies. Overall, skin testing is more sensitive and less costly than serologic anti-IgE antibody tests.[26]

Ibuprofen and paracetamol are the mainstay of symptomatic management in children younger than 2 years. In older patients and in the absence of tympanic perforation, topical analgesic preparations are useful. Evidence does not support routine use of decongestants and antihistamines.[28] The decision to use antibiotics in the treatment of OM is multifactorial. Generally, antibiotics are preserved for children younger than 2 years (10 days) or those older with toxic or severe symptoms or lack of proper access to health care or follow-ups (5–7 days). The antibiotic of choice is weight-based amoxicillin or Augmentin if the patient has taken a β-lactam within the month before the presentation of OM or in the presence of concurrent purulent conjunctivitis. In case of β-lactam allergy, macrolides or clindamycin are the antibiotics of choice but lacks coverage of *Haemophilus influenza* and one-third of pneumococcal pathogens.[29]

Sinusitis

CRS of the paranasal and nasal linings, by definition, lasts 12 weeks or longer.[30] The overlap of signs and symptoms, as well as the physical examination and radiographic findings with those of common upper respiratory tract infections has made the diagnosis of acute sinusitis a clinical challenge in pediatric patients.[31] Acute sinusitis is treated using antimicrobial agents, decongestants, and pain relief. There is no cure in most cases. The goal is to primarily relief symptoms, improve quality of life, and prevent complications.[32] In recurrent or complicated sinusitis, imaging such as coronal sinus computed tomography scans may be helpful. Bacterial culture and targeted antibiotic use are especially important in patients with chronic, refractory, and complicated cases and has proved to significantly decrease the mortality.[33] Sinus surgery may only be considered in complicated sinusitis in older patients and is generally contraindicated in younger patients with uncomplicated sinusitis.[34] There is a strong association between asthma and chronic rhinosinusitis at all ages, especially in presence of coexistent allergic rhinitis. Nasal discharge, facial pain/discomfort, nasal congestion, cough, and wheezing are the most common symptoms associated with chronic sinusitis in children. Chronic sinusitis may be an early sign of immunodeficiency or ciliary dysfunction.[35]

Multiple managements exist for CRS and may be used in combinations to address different subtypes. These include intranasal saline, intranasal and oral steroids, antibiotics, and antileukotriene agents. One of the determinants in the type of therapy for CRS is the presence of polyposis.[36,37] In the absence of such pathology, a combination of intranasal saline and steroids is the mainstay of management. The next step is to add oral steroids and a short course of antibiotics in refractory cases. Alternatively, experts recommend a long course of macrolides. The last resort, as mentioned earlier, will be endoscopic sinus surgery. Whatever the treatment, the importance of maintenance in management of patients with CRS should not be overlooked. Again, based the severity of the condition, maintenance regimens may range from a combination of intranasal saline and steroids to corticosteroid instillations.[35,36] Second-generation oral antihistamines, intranasal antihistamines, antileukotrienes (such as montelukast), and allergen immunomodulation may be used to overcome the symptoms of underlying allergic rhinitis.[24] In presence of nasal polyposis, the management of CRS is primarily similar to the nonpolyposis form, with the main goal of shrinking the polyp and getting relief from the blockage. Failure of these initial interventions will make the patient a candidate for surgery or biological therapy.[38] Currently only dupilumab is approved specifically for CRS with polyposis. In case of intolerance to aspirin, evidence supports aspirin desensitization and daily aspirin use.[39]

Chronic Cough

Cough may be classified as acute (<3 weeks), subacute (3–8 weeks), or chronic (>8 weeks). It is classified as *specific*, which is attributable to an underlying physiologic cause, or *nonspecific*, without an identifiable cause.[40] Specific cough most commonly results from asthma, bacterial bronchitis, bronchiectasis, mycoplasma, pertussis, and recurrent aspiration. One of the most common causes of chronic cough in children is postnasal drip, resulting in irritation of the upper airway. This cough may cause cough-variant asthma, allergic rhinitis, and rhinosinusitis.[41]

Less commonly, congenital anomalies, and neoplasia may cause chronic pediatric cough. Diagnosis is mainly through accurate history taking.[40,41]

The symptomatology of *specific* chronic cough includes productivity, wheezing, musculoskeletal chest pain, and hemoptysis. Chronic cough causes hypoxia, failure to thrive, feeding difficulties, and exertional dyspnea.[42] Physical examination may reveal chest wall abnormalities, digital clubbing, and abnormal lung auscultation. Chest radiograph and spirometry may aid in the workup. Chronic wet cough in a young child mainly points to an infectious pulmonary disease and should be treated with antibiotics. A chronic cough after an episode of choking while eating or while playing should raise suspicion for foreign body aspiration.[41] *Nonspecific cough*, on the other hand, is dry and nonproductive with normal physical examination, laboratory findings, and spirometry results. This type of pediatric cough should be managed by observation and will most like self-resolve. There is no evidence in support of efficacy of cough suppressants in management of chronic cough. In either form, environmental factors such as exposure to cigarette smoke should be assessed and eliminated.[40,43]

Atopic Dermatitis

Atopic dermatitis (AD) is the most common chronic inflammatory skin disease in childhood, affecting about 20% of children with highly pruritic rashes. Food allergens in particular have a major role in the pathogenesis of the disease especially early in life. There are numerous triggers and clinical symptoms for atopic dermatitis. A careful history and appropriate diagnostic testing will help in identifying the underlying cause.[44,45] AD is frequently found in association with respiratory allergy. The diagnosis is mainly based on clinical presentation with pruritus and chronic or relapsing eczematous dermatitis with typical distribution.[45] Skin hydration and use of topical antiinflammatory agents along with avoidance of allergenic triggers and skin irritants are the keys to management. Educating patients and parents is an essential part of AD treatment.[46] For patients failing on conventional symptom management, risks versus benefits of systemic treatment need to be discussed. AD is a frequently relapsing disease, and its prevalence has been increasing. Genetics, epigenetics, the host's environmental allergens, pharmacologic abnormalities, and immunologic factors are the interplays of complex pathogenesis of AD.[47]

Although AD is the most common chronic skin disease in children, it is important to consider differential diagnosis of a pruritic rash when managing it, especially if the response to treatment is suboptimal or presentation is atypical. Although cutaneous T-cell lymphoma/mycosis fungoides are rare, we need to bear them in mind while treating chronic skin disease. Primary treatment of AD consists of topical corticosteroids and emollients. The more severe the skin disease, the more potent the corticosteroids. Facial skin is susceptible to atrophy as a result of steroid therapy, and low-potency steroids should be used. For patients with moderate-to-severe disease and those with failed immunosuppressive treatment, dupilumab has shown promising results.[44,45,47]

Urticaria and Angioedema

Urticaria and angioedema are common skin disorders with clinical manifestations ranging from an isolated hive to life-threatening situation. Clinicians need to be able to characterize urticaria/angioedema by its type, chronicity, and pathogenesis.[48] Although determining the discrete cause of a chronic urticaria is rarely successful, a detailed history usually reveals causation of the acute urticaria/angioedema, and appropriate interventions can be instituted promptly. Although the treatment of chronic urticaria can be frustrating, symptoms can be adequately controlled until the swelling improves.[49] Although hereditary angioedema is a rare cause of recurrent angioedema, timely screening for it will protect these patients from severe morbidity and mortality.[50] Urticaria is either acute or chronic, with acute outbreaks resolving within 6 weeks. H1 antihistamines and H2 antihistamines are the mainstay of treatment of mild and moderate-to-severe modalities of urticarial, respectively. In presence of angioedema or failed H1/H2 treatments, a brief course of oral corticosteroids is recommended.[49,50]

Contact Dermatitis

Contact dermatitis (CD) has 2 forms of irritant and allergic. Although differentiating these two forms are very challenging, the key to differentiation is detailed medical history and assessment of exposures along with patch testing.[51] The main factor on managing allergic CD (ACD) is avoidance of the allergens. Gold standard for diagnosis of ACD at any age is patch test. Studies on induction of tolerance by targeting the immune mechanisms involved may lead to better treatment strategies especially with difficult-to-avoid allergens.[52] Emollients and moisturizers plus topical corticosteroids, separately or in combination, are the mainstay of CD treatment. Depending on the severity of the disease, a range of low to high potency corticosteroids will be used. Once more, clinician should avoid prescription of potent steroids for facial skin.[52,53]

Allergic Ophthalmopathy

One in every four children is diagnosed with some type of allergic disease, and in about one-third of them the only presentation is ocular involvement. Allergic ocular disorders in children are increasing in prevalence but our understanding of the pathogenesis of these disorders is still limited. Although the hallmark of allergic conjunctivitis is itching, infective conjunctivitis does not commonly manifest with pruritus. Unlike infection, allergic conjunctivitis generally has wax and waning symptoms over a long period of time coinciding with the environmental allergen (eg, seasonal pollens).[54–56]

The differential diagnosis of allergic ophthalmopathy (chronic allergic conjunctivitis) includes chronic conjunctival vascular injection due to the intense viewing of electronic devices, which may present itself as a *dry eye* disease. Dry eye symptoms may also be seen in patients taking systemic antihistamines. Topical steroids may increase the intraocular pressure (glaucoma) and should be used with caution in treating conjunctivitis in children. They also may exacerbate a herpes simplex virus keratoconjunctivitis.[54,56]

Drug Allergy

Although true drug hypersensitivity is relatively uncommon, its entire spectrum can be seen in children, even its most severe cutaneous or organ-specific types. Similar to adults, in most of the pediatric population, the drugs most frequently involved in hypersensitivity reactions are β-lactam antibiotics, nonsteroidal antiinflammatory drugs, acetaminophen, and other antibiotics.[57] The children who are labeled as being *allergic* to a medication will end up carrying this into their adulthood and are likely to be treated with alternative medications, which may be less effective, more toxic, or in case of antibiotics to spread certain types of drug-resistant bacteria.[58]

Latex Allergy

IgE-mediated allergy to natural rubber latex (NRL) emerged in the 1980s as an epidemic of anaphylaxis, allergies, and occupational asthma with NLR use in thousands of consumer and medical products. Clinical cross-reactivity of latex proteins with multiple foods, especially banana, avocado, and/or kiwi, may lead to clinical allergic responses in almost half of the latex-allergic subjects.[59] A small group of patients with fruit and vegetable allergies may develop allergic reactions from cross-reactivity to latex. Highest risk of latex allergy is seen in patients with spina bifida. Detailed medical history, physical examination, and patch testing are the keys to diagnosis, and up to 25% of serologic tests may produce false-positive results. Mainstem of treatment is avoidance of latex through *latex-safe precautions*.[60,61]

Insect Sting Allergy

Insect sting reactions in children are usually mild and frequently limited to the dermal layer (hives, angioedema). These patients have a very benign prognosis, but the more severe form has a 30% to 40% risk of recurrent anaphylaxis. These children should be provided with epinephrine autoinjector prescription while considering its risks and benefits. More than 95% protection against subsequent resting reactions is provided by venom immunotherapy over the course of 3 to 5 years, and this causes a milder reaction if any, despite the persistence of specific IgE.[62,63]

ANAPHYLAXIS

Anaphylaxis is an acute potentially life-threatening multisystem hypersensitivity reaction. It is caused by degranulation of mast cells and systemic release of IgE complexes in response to an allergen, including food, drugs, and insect bites.[64] The incidence of anaphylaxis reactions is estimated to be increasing in the United States, which is why it is important to be able to identify it appropriately and efficiently as to provide treatment in a timely fashion.[65]

Diagnosis includes recognition of sudden onset of signs and symptoms involving the skin and mucosal tissue (hives, pruritus or flushing, swollen lips-tongue-uvula), respiratory distress (nasal discharge, shortness of breath, wheezing), gastrointestinal symptoms (nausea, vomiting, diarrhea), and cardiac symptoms (palpitations, hypotension) within minutes to a few hours of exposure to an allergen. Prompt recognition and treatment are essential.[64,65] Management includes removal of offending agent; calling for assistance; intramuscular injection of epinephrine, 0.01 mg/kg, in the mid-outer thigh (maximum 0.15 mg in an infant, 0.3 mg in a child, and 0.5 mg in a teenager); and laying patient supine with elevation of lower extremities, supplemental oxygen, and intravenous (IV) fluids. In case of severe anaphylaxis reaction, intubation and CPR may be required in the event of cardiopulmonary compromise. Adjunctive therapy including H1 antihistamines, H2 antihistamines, bronchodilators, and glucocorticoids may be administered for additional symptom relief but should never be a substitute for epinephrine as the sole treatment.[65,66] Initial presentation of mild symptoms such as hives and cough should not trick the clinician in delaying a prompt intervention, as mild reactions have the potential to progress rapidly into life-threatening decompensation. If patients are not responding to initial therapy or seem to be deteriorating, they should immediately be admitted to the intensive care unit for closer monitoring. Once discharged, patients are advised to have an anaphylaxis emergency action plan, to carry at least one Epi pen at all time, and to wear medical identifiers. Health care workers should be trained to recognize early signs of anaphylaxis in community settings and the basic interventions such as use of Epi pen or calling for help while resuscitating. The best management is prevention. Patients with severe or uncontrolled asthma have higher risk of severe and fatal anaphylaxis. This underlines the importance of managing atopic and allergic comorbidities.[64–66]

DIAGNOSTICS
Laboratory Diagnosis

Although food antigen–specific IgG and IgG4 antibody levels are not predictive of food allergy, allergen-specific IgE antibodies may confirm allergic sensitization. Quantitative IgE antibody levels above a certain threshold are predictive and eliminate the need for further costly and time-consuming studies. The diagnostic threshold, however, is not similar across the populations, which questions the sensitivity and reliability of the test. On the other hand, successful immunotherapy is associated with high levels of allergen-specific IgG antibodies. Mast cell tryptase is used as a marker of mast cell activation during anaphylaxis. Its serum level equals less than 5 µg/L in healthy adults and is increased within 1 to 4 hours following onset of systemic anaphylaxis.[67,68]

In Vivo Testing

Skin testing is the preferred method for detection of IgE-mediated allergic reactions due to its objective endpoint. In addition, multiple sensitivities may be tested at once using skin testing. Most patients with asthma and allergic rhinitis have positive skin tests. This test, however, does not show high specificity, as asymptomatic subjects also test positive sometimes. Therefore, the diagnosis should mainly be based on clinical presentation. In terms of sensitivity, some patients with allergic rhinitis have negative skin and in vitro tests for the relevant allergens. In case of nasal allergy, however, a positive nasal challenge confirms the disease. Regardless of the allergen, positive skin tests are most common in the third decade and least common in pediatric and geriatric populations. Prick/puncture skin tests have lower sensitivity compared with the intradermal tests with the same extract concentration.[67-69]

MANAGEMENT
Prevention

Allergic sensitization usually initiates in a mild form in early childhood, although it can arise at any age. Environmental allergens induce allergen-specific IgE; their presence is often transient and mostly resolves spontaneously. Persistence and consolidation of such reactions leads to the development of allergies. For the same reason, although atopic sensitization is an important risk factor for allergic disorders such as asthma, a small subset of atopic individuals will develop persistent asthma, which indicates the importance of other cofactors involved.[2,6]

The modern environment has compound social, cultural, and economic risk factors for development of allergy. Strategies to effectively overcome these risk factors present even greater challenges. There is little information on why allergies are less common in developing countries and have the highest rate in countries with westernized lifestyle. In particular, improved hygiene, less exposure to microbial organisms, changes in diet (eating less fish and vegetables), less exposure to sunlight (reduced ultraviolet and therefore reduced vitamin D), and possibly increased use of antibiotics are thought to be the main factors contributing specifically to an increase in food allergy.[1,6,27]

Environmental Control

Exposure avoidance measures can significantly reduce symptoms and medication requirements. Based on NAEPP-EPR 3 guidelines, clinicians should identify allergen exposures, assess specific sensitivities to indoor allergens using skin or laboratory testing, and implement environmental controls to minimize exposure. Chronic allergic symptoms, including asthma, allergic rhinitis, and atopic dermatitis, should be assessed by exposure and sensitivity tests for all potential indoor allergens. Avoidance will be the first-line therapy for patients with positive indoor allergen workup. Moreover, a comprehensive specific environmental control strategy should be implemented based on sensitivity test results. Such strategies aim to downregulate IgE receptors, halt mast cell survival, decrease allergen uptake by B cells, and block Th2 cytokine expression by mast cells. Novel anti-IgE therapies are currently the main focus of research and are believed to be the most beneficial.[10,11]

Management of Food Allergy

Consistent with general environmental control measures, current management of food allergy mainly involves dietary avoidance. Although this may seem an easy task, there are several concerns that need to be sufficiently addressed by the clinician. Most importantly, accidental ingestions are not uncommon; this highlights the importance of educating the patients and their caregivers on how to read and interpret product labels to successfully identify and eliminate food allergens. It also shows the importance of patient education on how to recognize and treat such allergic reactions. Moreover, such diets have potential social, psychological, financial, and nutritional burdens for families. Children with food allergies may have inadequate nutrient intake and poor growth and may need appropriate substitute foods and formulas.[13-15,20]

Immunotherapy

Alteration of humoral and cellular immune responses is a very effective treatment modality for the pediatric patient with allergic rhinitis, stinging insect allergy, and allergic asthma. Immune-modulating therapeutics are administered through different routes just like any other medication. However, compared with the subcutaneous immunotherapy, sublingual agents have been associated with much smaller risk of systemic reactions. Oral immunotherapy has shown promising results and is a subject of wide research in contemporary food allergy treatment.[1,2,68,69]

CLINICS CARE POINTS

- Allergic rhinitis requires management over a long period of time with allergen avoidance, pharmacotherapy (glucocorticoid nasal sprays and second generation antihistamines), and, in refractory cases, immunotherapy.

- Avoidance of irritants is crucial in the treatment of dry skin and cCD. Use of moisturizers and topical corticosteroids (systemic for face) are the mainstays of dry skin and cCD treatments, respectively.

- Although skin tests and IgE levels confirm sensitization, the gold standard for diagnosing food allergy remains to be an oral food challenge.

- Ibuprofen and paracetamol are the mainstays of symptomatic management of OM in children younger than 2 years. In older patients and in the absence of tympanic perforation, topical analgesic preparations are useful. Evidence does not support routine use of decongestants and antihistamines.

- Intranasal saline, intranasal and oral steroids, antibiotics, and antileukotriene agents can be used in combination in management of chronic rhinosinusitis.

- Primary treatment of atopic dermatitis consists of topical corticosteroids and emollients. The more severe the skin disease, the more potent the corticosteroids.

- Anaphylaxis management includes removal of offending agent; intramuscular injection of epinephrine, 0.01 mg/kg, in the mid-outer thigh; and laying patient supine with elevation of lower extremities, supplemental oxygen, and IV fluids.

DISCLOSURE

The authors declare that they have no relevant or material financial interests that relate to the research described in this article.

REFERENCES

1. Galli SJ, Tsai M. IgE and mast cells in allergic disease. Nat Med 2012;18(5): 693–704.
2. Chaplin DD. Overview of the immune response. J Allergy Clin Immunol 2010; 125(2 Suppl 2):S3–23.
3. Murdoch JR, Lloyd CM. Chronic inflammation and asthma. Mutat Res 2010; 690(1–2):24–39.
4. Wu HJ, Wu E. The role of gut microbiota in immune homeostasis and autoimmunity. Gut Microbes 2012;3(1):4–14.
5. Patel NP, Prizment AE, Thyagarajan B, et al. Urban vs rural residency and allergy prevalence among adult women: Iowa Women's Health Study. Ann Allergy Asthma Immunol 2018;120(6):654.e1.
6. Doll RJ, Joseph NI, McGarry D, et al. Epidemiology of allergic diseases. In: Mahmoudi M, Craig T, Ledford D, editors. Allergy and asthma: the basics to best practices. Cham (Switzerland): Springer International Publishing; 2019. p. 31–51.
7. Lemke M, Hartert TV, Gebretsadik T, et al. Relationship of secondhand smoke and infant lower respiratory tract infection severity by familial atopy status. Ann Allergy Asthma Immunol 2013;110(6):433–7.
8. Sicherer SH, Eggleston PA. Environmental Allergens. In: Lieberman P, Anderson JA, editors. Allergic diseases: diagnosis and treatment. Totowa (NJ): Humana Press; 2007. p. 39–50.
9. Reinmuth-Selzle K, Kampf CJ, Lucas K, et al. Air Pollution and Climate Change Effects on Allergies in the Anthropocene: Abundance, Interaction, and Modification of Allergens and Adjuvants. Environ Sci Technol 2017;51(8):4119–41.
10. Acevedo N, Zakzuk J, Caraballo L. House Dust Mite Allergy Under Changing Environments. Allergy Asthma Immunol Res 2019;11(4):450–09.
11. Ahluwalia SK, Matsui EC. Indoor Environmental Interventions for Furry Pet Allergens, Pest Allergens, and Mold: Looking to the Future. J Allergy Clin Immunol Pract 2018;6(1):9–19.
12. Valenta R, Hochwallner H, Linhart B, et al. Food allergies: the basics. Gastroenterology 2015;148(6):1120.e4.
13. Labrosse R, Graham F, Caubet JC. Non-IgE-mediated gastrointestinal food allergies in children: an update. Nutrients 2020;12(7):2086.
14. Dhar S, Srinivas SM. Food allergy in atopic dermatitis. Indian J Dermatol 2016; 61(6):645–8.
15. Hochwallner H, Schulmeister U, Swoboda I, et al. Cow's milk allergy: from allergens to new forms of diagnosis, therapy and prevention. Methods 2014;66(1): 22–33.
16. Meyer R, Chebar Lozinsky A, Fleischer DM, et al. Diagnosis and management of Non-IgE gastrointestinal allergies in breastfed infants—An EAACI Position Paper. Allergy 2020;75(1):14–32.
17. Dellon ES. Eosinophilic esophagitis: diagnostic tests and criteria. Curr Opin Gastroenterol 2012;28(4):382–8.
18. Kashyap RR, Kashyap RS. Oral Allergy Syndrome: An Update for Stomatologists. J Allergy (Cairo) 2015;2015:543928.
19. Sussman G, Sussman A, Sussman D. Oral allergy syndrome. CMAJ 2010; 182(11):1210–1.
20. Calvani M, Bianchi A, Reginelli C, et al. Oral food challenge. Medicina (Kaunas) 2019 Sep 27;55(10):651.

21. Dykewicz MS, Wallace DV, Amrol DJ, et al. Rhinitis 2020: A practice parameter update. J Allergy Clin Immunol 2020;146(4):721–67.
22. Wheatley LM, Togias A. Clinical practice. Allergic rhinitis. N Engl J Med 2015; 372(5):456–63.
23. Varshney J, Varshney H. Allergic Rhinitis: an Overview. Indian J Otolaryngol Head Neck Surg 2015;67(2):143–9.
24. Small P, Keith PK, Kim H. Allergic rhinitis. Allergy Asthma Clin Immunol 2018; 14(2):51.
25. Schilder AG, Chonmaitree T, Cripps AW, et al. Otitis media. Nat Rev Dis Primers 2016;2:16063.
26. Zernotti ME, Pawankar R, Ansotegui I, et al. Otitis media with effusion and atopy: is there a causal relationship? World Allergy Organ J 2017;10(1):37.
27. Ledford DK, Lockey RF. Asthma and comorbidities. Curr Opin Allergy Clin Immunol 2013;13(1):78–86.
28. Sjoukes A, Venekamp RP, van de Pol AC, et al. Paracetamol (acetaminophen) or non-steroidal anti-inflammatory drugs, alone or combined, for pain relief in acute otitis media in children. Cochrane Database Syst Rev 2016;12:CD011534.
29. Darrow DH, Dash N, Derkay CS. Otitis media: concepts and controversies. Curr Opin Otolaryngol Head Neck Surg 2003;11(6):416–23.
30. Orlandi RR, Kingdom TT, Hwang PH, et al. International Consensus Statement on Allergy and Rhinology: Rhinosinusitis. Int Forum Allergy Rhinol 2016;6(Suppl 1): S22–209.
31. Shaikh N, Hoberman A, Kearney DH, et al. Signs and symptoms that differentiate acute sinusitis from viral upper respiratory tract infection. Pediatr Infect Dis J 2013;32(10):1061–5.
32. Suh JD, Kennedy DW. Treatment Options for Chronic Rhinosinusitis. Proc Am Thorac Soc 2011;8(1):132–40.
33. Meltzer EO, Hamilos DL, Hadley JA, et al. Rhinosinusitis: Establishing definitions for clinical research and patient care. Otolaryngol Head Neck Surg 2004;131(6 Suppl):S1–62.
34. Badr DT, Gaffin JM, Phipatanakul W. Pediatric Rhinosinusitis. Curr Treat Options Allergy 2016;3(3):268–81.
35. Scadding GK. Rhinitis and Sinusitis. Clin Respir Med 2008;409–23.
36. Cain RB, Lal D. Update on the management of chronic rhinosinusitis. Infect Drug Resist 2013;6:1–14.
37. Meltzer EO, Hamilos DL. Rhinosinusitis diagnosis and management for the clinician: a synopsis of recent consensus guidelines. Mayo Clin Proc 2011;86(5): 427–43.
38. Stevens WW, Schleimer RP, Kern RC. Chronic Rhinosinusitis with Nasal Polyps. J Allergy Clin Immunol Pract 2016;4(4):565–72.
39. Patel GB, Kern RC, Bernstein JA, et al. Current and Future Treatments of Rhinitis and Sinusitis. J Allergy Clin Immunol Pract 2020;8(5):1522–31.
40. Alsubaie H, Al-Shamrani A, Alharbi AS, et al. Clinical practice guidelines: Approach to cough in children: The official statement endorsed by the Saudi Pediatric Pulmonology Association (SPPA). Int J Pediatr Adolesc Med 2015;2(1): 38–43.
41. Kantar A. Phenotypic presentation of chronic cough in children. J Thorac Dis 2017;9(4):907–13.
42. Marchant JM, Masters IB, Taylor SM, et al. Utility of signs and symptoms of chronic cough in predicting specific cause in children. Thorax 2006;61(8):694–8.

43. De Blasio F, Virchow JC, Polverino M, et al. Cough management: a practical approach. Cough 2011;7(1):7.
44. Kapur S, Watson W, Carr S. Atopic dermatitis. Allergy Asthma Clin Immunol 2018; 14(Suppl 2):52.
45. Lyons JJ, Milner JD, Stone KD. Atopic dermatitis in children: clinical features, pathophysiology, and treatment. Immunol Allergy Clin North Am 2015;35(1): 161–83.
46. Boguniewicz M, Leung DY. The ABC's of managing patients with severe atopic dermatitis. J Allergy Clin Immunol 2013;132(2):511.e5.
47. Stofella Sodre C, Ferreira DC, Vieira MS, et al. Clinical oral profile of pediatric patients with atopic dermatitis: A cross-sectional study. Oral Dis 2020. https://doi. org/10.1111/odi.13721.
48. Kanani A, Betschel SD, Warrington R. Urticaria and angioedema. Allergy Asthma Clin Immunol 2018;14(Suppl 2):59.
49. Schaefer P. Acute and Chronic Urticaria: Evaluation and Treatment. Am Fam Physician 2017;95(11):717–24.
50. Zuraw BL. 52 - Urticaria and angioedema. In: Leung DYM, et al, editors. Pediatric allergy: principles and practice. 3rd edition. London: Elsevier; 2016. p. 458–66.e3.
51. Owen JL, Vakharia PP, Silverberg JI. The role and diagnosis of allergic contact dermatitis in patients with atopic dermatitis. Am J Clin Dermatol 2018;19(3): 293–302.
52. Uter W, Werfel T, White IR, et al. Contact allergy: a review of current problems from a clinical perspective. Int J Environ Res Public Health 2018;15(6):1108.
53. Rathi SK, D'Souza P. Rational and ethical use of topical corticosteroids based on safety and efficacy. Indian J Dermatol 2012;57(4):251–9.
54. Azari AA, Arabi A. Conjunctivitis: A Systematic Review. J Ophthalmic Vis Res 2020;15(3):372–95.
55. Azari AA, Barney NP. Conjunctivitis: a systematic review of diagnosis and treatment. JAMA 2013;310(16):1721–9.
56. Vazirani J, Shukla S, Chhawchharia R, et al. Allergic conjunctivitis in children: current understanding and future perspectives. Curr Opin Allergy Clin Immunol 2020;20(5):507–15.
57. Warrington R, Silviu-Dan F, Wong T. Drug allergy. Allergy Asthma Clin Immunol 2018;14(Suppl 2):60.
58. Stone SF, Phillips EJ, Wiese MD, et al. Immediate-type hypersensitivity drug reactions. Br J Clin Pharmacol 2014;78(1):1–13.
59. Nucera E, Aruanno A, Rizzi A, et al. Latex Allergy: Current Status and Future Perspectives. J Asthma Allergy 2020;13:385–98.
60. Kurup VP, Sussman GL, Yeang HY, et al. Specific IgE response to purified and recombinant allergens in latex allergy. Clin Mol Allergy 2005;3:11.
61. Wu M, McIntosh J, Liu J. Current prevalence rate of latex allergy: Why it remains a problem? J Occup Health 2016;58(2):138–44.
62. Pesek RD, Lockey RF. Management of insect sting hypersensitivity: an update. Allergy Asthma Immunol Res 2013;5(3):129–37.
63. Przybilla B, Rueff F. Insect stings: clinical features and management. Dtsch Arztebl Int 2012;109(13):238–48.
64. Cardona V, Ansotegui IJ, Ebisawa M, et al. World allergy organization anaphylaxis guidance 2020. World Allergy Organ J 2020;13(10):100472.
65. Turner PJ, Jerschow E, Umasunthar T, et al. Fatal Anaphylaxis: Mortality Rate and Risk Factors. J Allergy Clin Immunol Pract 2017;5(5):1169–78.

66. Jarvinen KM, Celestin J. Anaphylaxis avoidance and management: educating patients and their caregivers. J Asthma Allergy 2014;7:95–104.
67. Ansotegui IJ, Melioli G, Canonica GW, et al. IgE allergy diagnostics and other relevant tests in allergy, a World Allergy Organization position paper. World Allergy Organ J 2020;13(2):100080.
68. Popov TA, Passalacqua G, González-Díaz SN, et al. Medical devices in allergy practice. World Allergy Organ J 2020;13(10):100466.
69. Pfaar O, Bachert C, Bufe A, et al. Guideline on allergen-specific immunotherapy in IgE-mediated allergic diseases: S2k Guideline of the German Society for Allergology and Clinical Immunology (DGAKI), the Society for Pediatric Allergy and Environmental Medicine (GPA), the Medical Association of German Allergologists (AeDA), the Austrian Society for Allergy and Immunology (ÖGAI), the Swiss Society for Allergy and Immunology (SGAI), the German Society of Dermatology (DDG), the German Society of Oto- Rhino-Laryngology, Head and Neck Surgery (DGHNO-KHC), the German Society of Pediatrics and Adolescent Medicine (DGKJ), the Society for Pediatric Pneumology (GPP), the German Respiratory Society (DGP), the German Association of ENT Surgeons (BV-HNO), the Professional Federation of Paediatricians and Youth Doctors (BVKJ), the Federal Association of Pulmonologists (BDP) and the German Dermatologists Association (BVDD). Allergo J Int 2014;23(8):282–319.

Moving?

Make sure your subscription moves with you!

To notify us of your new address, find your **Clinics Account Number** (located on your mailing label above your name), and contact customer service at:

Email: journalscustomerservice-usa@elsevier.com

800-654-2452 (subscribers in the U.S. & Canada)
314-447-8871 (subscribers outside of the U.S. & Canada)

Fax number: 314-447-8029

Elsevier Health Sciences Division
Subscription Customer Service
3251 Riverport Lane
Maryland Heights, MO 63043

*To ensure uninterrupted delivery of your subscription, please notify us at least 4 weeks in advance of move.